1735

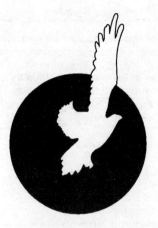

A Sourcebook for Helping People in Spiritual Emergency

by
Emma Bragdon, Ph.D.

Lightening Up Press
California

copyright © 1988 by Emma Bragdon

All rights reserved. No part of this work may be reproduced or
transmitted in any form or by any means, electronic or mechanical,
including photcopying and recording, or by any information storage
or retreival system, except as may be expressly permitted by the 1976
Copyright Act or in writing from the publisher. Requests for such
permissions should be addressed to: Lightening Up Press, 885 No. San
Antonio Road, Suite 'R', Los Altos, California 94022.

Library of Congress Cataloging in Publication Data

Bragdon, Emma, 1946-
Sourcebook for Helping People
in Spiritual Emergency
Bibliography: p. 257
1. Psychology 2. Religion 3. Consciousness
I. Title

LC# 88-092082

Printed in the United States of America

The article entitled "Mysticism Goes Mainstream" by Andrew Greeley
was originally published by American Health Partners in 1987. It is
reprinted by permission of Andrew Greeley.

Jossey-Bass, Inc. originally published the article "Soteria: An Alternative for Schizophrenics" by Loren Mosher and Alma Menn in 1979 in
New Directions for Mental Health Services. Permission to reprint this
article came from the authors and Jossey-Bass, Inc., and Grune and
Stratton who published a version of this article edited by Masserman
in 1982 in *Current Psychiatric Therapies, Vol. 21*.

The Spiritual Emergence Network gave permission to reprint the
article "Forms of Spiritual Emergency" initially published in the
Spiritual Emergency Network Newsletter in 1985.

Permission to reprint the review article "Schizophrenics for whom
Phenothiazines are Contraindicated or Unnecessary" (1971) was given
by Dr. Julian Silverman.

ISBN 0-9620960-0-8

Dedication

This book is dedicated to the people who have been Helpers in my spiritual awakening. In the most general sense, this includes all sentient beings. For the Buddhists say, each sentient being has at one time been my mother. In a more specific way, the book is dedicated to Suzuki Roshi, Harry Roberts, Marilyn Youngbird, and my family. These people have supported my spiritual emergence in profound ways for which I am deeply grateful.

Acknowledgements

The idea for this sourcebook came to me because I have been so profoundly inspired by the work of Stanislav and Christina Grof.

I want to acknowledge my dear friends - William Brater, Laura Sosnowski, Mackie Ramsay, and Judith Whitman-Small for their unwavering support during this project. Enthusiasm, uplifting energy and editorial suggestions came from Nikki Kester, Jamie Baraz, Betty Herring, Sandra Glickman, Elizabeth Campbell, Jill Mellick, Val Young, David Lukoff, Ronda Dave, Theresa Muñoz, Susanna Davila and Nancy Rosser-Hutchins. These people were essential to the completion of this manual.

Book design and typesetting was done by John Verducci at AlphaGraphics of Los Altos. The cover was designed and produced by Barnett Associates of Aptos, California. The art was directed by Dan Drabek. The book was printed by Delta Lithograph Company of Los Angeles. I am grateful for the technical assistance and personal care in business which greeted me at every turn.

My clients and friends have unwittingly been a wealth of support to my increased knowledge of the spiritual emergence process. I thank them for their difficulties, their successes, their aspirations, and their willingness to share so deeply with me.

Table of Contents

Table of Contents

Table of Contents

Table of Contents

List of Tables

This book is a section of my Ph.D. dissertation, **A Sourcebook for Helping people in Spiritual Emergency**, completed in March, 1987, at the Institute for Transpersonal Psychology in Menlo Park, California.

Note that in all case examples, names, and other identifiable details have been altered to protect confidentiality.

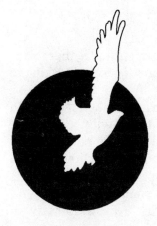

Introduction ————————————————————

The Sourcebook and
The Spiritual Emergence Network

This sourcebook was written as a guideline for professionals and paraprofessionals in the field of human services on helping someone in spiritual emergency. Spiritual emergency is a new diagnostic category which refers to profound disorientation and instability that sometimes accompanies intense spiritual experience. It appears as an acute psychotic episode lasting between minutes and weeks, and eventually having a positive transformative outcome (Dabrowski, 1964; Grof,1985; Lukoff, 1986). People in such a crisis have needs for care that are usually unavailable from therapists, doctors, or in hospitals dealing with more typical psychoses.

The Sourcebook

This sourcebook is written for professional therapists, pastoral counselors, paraprofessional people working in crisis situations, and students in training for these positions. It will also be useful to leaders and teachers in spiritual communities who are faced with the care of laypeople in personal crises catalyzed, in part, by their spiritual practice. The sourcebook is written from a transpersonal orientation. Transpersonal, as used in this sourcebook means related to experiences that are beyond normal ego states [See Appendix E for a glossary of terms].

The intended audience for this edition of the sourcebook includes the Regional Coordinators and Helpers of the Spiritual Emergence Network, (SEN). SEN is a networking and referral organization which brings people who need support in their spiritual emergence together with health care workers qualified to provide that support.

Helpers are professionals and paraprofessionals who act as companions and guides to persons in spiritual emergency. There are currently 1200 Helpers, and about 40 Regional Coordinators serving in SEN all over the world. They have a common understanding of spiritual emergence as the process of personal awakening into a level of perceiving and functioning that is beyond normal ego functions. Many have had some experience with the work of Stan and Christina Grof who founded SEN.

Helpers represent a diverse spectrum of professionals and paraprofessionals, each bringing different skills and attitudes to their work with clients. These Helpers need a manual such as this because they have the most interaction with people in spiritual emergency. Helpers are also invited to evaluate this sourcebook in preparation for an edition oriented toward a larger audience.

This current edition of the sourcebook is designed to provide those now involved with SEN and those who may be doing similar work outside of SEN with a shared understanding of:

1. The definition of spiritual emergence/ emergency/ experience.
2. The difference between spiritual emergence phenomena and the symptoms of psychosis.
3. Clinical skills needed to help people in spiritual emergency.
4. The environment best suited to caring for people in spiritual emergency.

As understanding of these concepts and skills is gained a vocabulary will emerge to facilitate communication both within SEN and with other professional and paraprofessional communities.

Another important function of this sourcebook is to teach Helpers the skills to deal with spiritual emergency. The most needed information for Helpers will be:

1. Forms of spiritual emergency.
2. Psycho-social stressors.
3. Criteria for identifying spiritual emergency.

4. First interactions with people in crisis.
5. Elements of a safe environment.
6. Skills for grounding.
7. Skills for changing obsolete response patterns.
8. Supporting spiritual emergence.
9. Helper competencies.
10. Referrals.
11. A reading list about the phenomena of spiritual emergence.

Where appropriate, these subjects are first outlined to serve as a checklist and then explained in depth. This design should facilitate learning about the process of helping someone in spiritual emergency and provide a quick reference tool for use in a clinical setting.

The sourcebook has been designed to identify resources Helpers are already using. Questionnaires are provided in chapters 5 and 6 to help the reader identify his or her own resources as a Helper and the resources of the community. These questionnaires could also be used to stimulate discussion in groups learning about spiritual emergency as well as to help individuals clarify how they would deal with clients, students, and friends in spiritual crisis.

Spiritual Emergence Network

SEN was started in 1980 at Esalen Institute by Stanislav and Christina Grof. In 1984 it was moved to the Institute of Transpersonal Psychology (ITP) in Menlo Park, California, under the supervision of Susanna Davila, the head of ITP's Transpersonal Counseling Center.

SEN is currently increasing its focus on recognizing and responding to people in spiritual emergency. SEN publishes a newsletter and journal containing articles of interest to people who support the network and periodically gives related workshops and seminars. An annual conference for invited participants is hosted by Esalen Institute for leaders in the field of working with people in spiritual emergency. These conferences represent the leading edge of current thinking, research, and clinical work in this field and help to reinforce the community spirit within the network. Chapter 9, "Suggestions for the Future of SEN," reflects on future plans for the development of SEN.

Many of the ideas in this sourcebook were introduced at the Esalen conferences. Guests at the first conference held in May, 1985, were informed at the time of their invitation that one outcome of the conference would be ideas for a book to teach people how to handle spiritual emergencies. Guests at the second conference held in October, 1985, were not specifically asked for contributions although they were aware that the book was in process. The people who participated in these conferences are listed in Appendix D of the manual.

Other ideas in this sourcebook were taken from materials listed in the References and from my personal experience.

About the Author

I have been involved in spiritual and transpersonal study for 20 years. I completed my doctoral studies at the Institute for Transpersonal Psychology and an internship at its Transpersonal Counseling Center. I am currently in private practice in Los Altos and Soquel, California. This manual is a section of my dissertation. Before coming to the Institute, I was in private practice as a Reichian bodyworker and teacher of co-counseling. I have been involved in the practice of hatha yoga and meditation for most of my adult life. I lived within the San Francisco Zen Center community for 4 years, studied intensively in the Ananda Community for 3 years, and am currently involved with the Subud Fellowship. My son's four year participation with the Rudolf Steiner Waldorf School system has also contributed to my knowledge of spiritual communities.

Throughout my life, I have been witness to or "Helper" for people in spiritual emergency. The most impressive experience of this nature was my mother's crisis reported in Chapter 7, Case Study. While participating in spiritual communities I have observed many spiritual emergencies. In my clinical practice, I have been given the opportunity to work with people in spiritual crises.

Spiritual Emergence and Psychology

The area of spiritual emergence is relatively new to western psychology. Even though spiritual emergence is increasingly apparent on a global scale (reviewed in chapter 8); the recognition of and response to spiritual emergence in professional circles are just beginning. There are few people writing, speaking, or doing research on the topic; few funds for research; little promotion for developing the skills of being a Helper, and few centers for people in spiritual emergency in need of round-the-clock care.

Credibility has been given to the area of spiritual emergence by studies such as those by Ring(1984) and Greeley(1987) which show that a majority of Americans have had spiritual experiences. Such statistical studies enhance the acceptance by the psychological community of spiritual emergency as a diagnostic category.

At this time, a common language is needed with which to speak about spiritual emergence phenomena. We need greater understanding of how to help. We need to enhance our skills as Helpers. This sourcebook is intended to contribute in each of these areas.

I welcome your feedback on this manual. I am particularly interested in what information has been **useful** to you, what has been **unclear** or inadequately defined, and what **suggestions** you have for additions. You can contact me c/o SEN, 250 Oak Grove Ave, Menlo Park, CA, 94025. Thankyou.

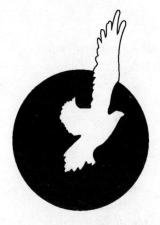

Chapter One ————————————

What are Spiritual Emergence, Spiritual Experience and Spiritual Emergency?

What is spiritual emergence? What happens to people who experience it? How many have had this experience? How does it relate to spiritual experience? How does it differ from spiritual emergency? What are the possible forms of spiritual emergence? How has spiritual emergency been confused with more typical psychopathological disorders?

This chapter addresses these questions and gives a theoretical foundation that will be the basis for later chapters on care-giving to persons in spiritual emergency.

Spiritual Emergence

> *"Spiritual emergence is a kind of birth pang in which you yourself go through to a fuller life, a deeper life, in which some areas in your life that were not yet encompassed by this fullness of life are now integrated or called to be integrated or challenged to be integrated ...Breakthroughs are often very painful, often acute and dramatic break-throughs (happen) on all levels: what we call material, spiritual, bodily-all levels."*

> *(Brother David Steindl-Rast, 1985)*

Spiritual emergence is the process of personal awakening into a level of perceiving and functioning which is beyond normal ego functioning. The process may at first include any of the following phenomena: out-of-body experiences, occult phenomena, precog-nition, clairvoyance, astral travel, and perception of auras. At its peak, spiritual emergence is the experience of the ultimate unity of all things, a mystical experience, a merging with the Divine which transcends verbal description. Among the positive effects of this process are increased creativity, feelings of peace, and an expanded sense of compassion.

Spiritual emergence processes are part of the passage of human development into transpersonal realms. Ken Wilber explores these in his theory of the spectrum of consciousness (1980), which illustrates the movement from prepersonal to transpersonal consciousness throughout the life cycle. His definition of transpersonal

10

levels, drawn from ancient eastern religious texts as well as more modern studies, gives us a vocabulary to communicate about levels of consciousness found in spiritual emergence.

Below is Wilber's diagram of the complete life cycle:

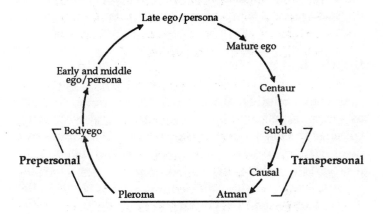

The Complete Life Cycle

Wilber's first level is the 'pleroma', where one perceives oneself as indistinguishable from one's mother. From here, one moves through the prepersonal levels to early, middle, and late ego development. During ego development, one realizes one's independence, perceives the world in concrete terms, and becomes increasingly capable of ordering one's life with the self-discipline necessary for financial and social survival.

A still higher order of self-organization is the Centauric self. This is the level of self-actualization, when one has successfully integrated body and mind. After this level has been fully reached, it is possible to actualize still higher levels of consciousness (the Subtle, Causal, and Atman), realms which bring one into more direct and conscious relationship to one's own life force.

Subtle Realm

In the Low -Subtle realm one will have experiences such as seeing auras, traveling out-of -body, and witnessing psi phenomena. To enter this plane of consciousness, one has to "more-or-less master psychic phenomena, or at least certain of them" (Wilber,1980, p.67). These psychic phenomena include clairvoyance, clairsentience, the ability to manifest psychokinetic phenomena, and the ability to heal through 'laying on of hands' or the like.

On entering the High-Subtle realm, one experiences "high religious intuition and literal inspiration...symbolic visions...audible illuminations and brightness upon brightness; it is the realm of higher presences, guides, angelic beings..." (ibid., p.68). Gopi Krishna, who experienced this realm as a result of his meditation practice, described it in the following manner :

> *Suddenly, with a roar like that of a waterfall, I felt*
> *a stream of liquid light entering my brain through*
> *the spinal cord...The illumination grew brighter*

and brighter, the roaring louder. I experienced a rocking sensation and then felt myself slipping out of my body, entirely enveloped in a halo of light. It is impossible to describe the experience accurately. I felt the point of consciousness that was myself growing wider, surrounded by waves of light. It grew wider and wider, spreading outward while the body, normally the immediate object of its perception, appeared to have receded into the distance until I became entirely unconscious of it. I was now all consciousness, without any outline, without any idea of a corporeal appendage, without any feeling or sensation coming from the senses, immersed in a sea of light simultaneously conscious and aware of every point, spread out, as it were, in all directions without any barrier or material obstruction. I was no longer myself, or to be more accurate, no longer as I knew myself to be, a small point of awareness confined in a body, but instead was a vast circle of consciousness in which the body was but a point, bathed in light and in a state of exaltation and happiness impossible to describe.

(Gopi Krishna, 1971, p.12-13)

Causal Realm

In the Low-Causal realm one's identification condenses and dissolves into God and becomes God (Wilber,1980, p.71). In the High-Causal realm, conscious-ness expands still further to include the knowing of "formlessness," the "ecstasy of the void" (ibid., p.73). Following is an example of Causal realm experience:

> *Soul and mind instantly lost their physical bondage...In my intense awareness I knew that never before had I been fully alive. My sense of identity was no longer narrowly confined to a body...People on distant streets seemed to be moving gently over my own remote periphery...An oceanic joy broke upon the endless calm shores of my soul.*

> *(Yogananda, 1969, p.149-150)*

People who have integrated experiences of the Causal realm into their lives often become spiritual teachers. In their presence one feels the deep wisdom they have attained and the loving compassion which they freely give to all.

> *There is no more of the alternation of pain and pleasure, only a constant and pervasive joy...(He)/ She) reflects an inner discipline and an inner peace—through a relaxed body and harmonious coordination, and through patience, confidence, clear thinking, and an unselfish attention to the needs of others.*
> *(Rama et al., 1976, p. 205-206)*

Atman

The final state of Atman, or Ultimate Unity, is defined thus:

> *This is not itself a state apart from other states; it is not an altered state; it is not a special state-it is rather the suchness of all states...this is the radically*

> *perfect integration of all prior levels-gross, subtle
> and causal, which, now of themselves, continue to
> arise moment to moment in an iridescent play of
> mutual interpenetration...Consciousness
> henceforth operates, not on the world, but only as
> the entire World Process, integrating and
> interpenetrating all levels, realms, and planes,
> high or low, sacred or profane.*

> *(Wilber, 1980, p. 74)*

This is a rare state of consciousness. No one, as yet, has devised a way to measure how many people have achieved it. Yet, however extraordinary it is, it has been described in the literature of ancient world religions as well as in modern anthologies (Vaughan and Walsh, 1980; White, 1984).

Proof of Subtle and Causal experience is characterized by an "appreciation of the wholistic, unitive, integrated nature of the universe and one's unity with it." (Vaughan and Walsh, 1980, p.47). The people who have experienced this greater reality and integrated it into their lives "are likely to be better educated, more economically successful, less racist, and substantially higher on scores of psychological well-being." (Allison, 1967; Greeley, 1975; Hood, 1974, 1976; Thomas and Cooper, 1977)

More substantiation of the positive effect of spiritual emergence on people comes from the work of Ring (1980,1984) who notes that the experience of physically dying for a brief time serves as a catalyst for rapid spiritual growth. After a near-death experience (NDE), people manifest a particular change in their world view:

15

After NDEs, individuals tend to show greater appreciation for life and more concern and love for their fellow humans while their interest in personal status and material possessions wanes. Most NDErs also state that they live afterward with a heightened sense of spiritual purpose.

Following an NDE, people generally exhibit;

1. *A tendency to characterize oneself as spiritual rather than religious per se.*

2. *A feeling of being inwardly close to God.*

3. *A de-emphasis of the formal aspects of religious life and worship.*

4. *A conviction that there is life after death, regardless of religious belief.*

5. *An openness to the doctrine of reincarnation (and a general sympathy toward Eastern religions).*

6. *A belief in the essential underlying unity of all religions.*

7. *A desire for a universal religion embracing all humanity.*

(Ring, 1984, p.142-146)

People who have had near-death experiences, NDErs, number at least 8 million in North America according to a 1982 Gallup survey. There is evidence in Ring's book (1984) suggesting that more and more people will be introduced to the Subtle and Causal levels of experience because of the improvements in our resuscitation technology that allow people to physically die for a short period and then be brought back to life.

Anaesthetics, especially ketamine, can promote NDE-like experiences (Rogo, 1984). Psychotropic drugs such as LSD and MDMA (Ecstasy) produce the phenomena of transpersonal experience (Grof, 1980; Greer, 1983; Strassman, 1984). The influences of these medical and pharmaceutical experiences on our lives (and other psycho-social factors discussed in chapters 2 and 8), all contribute to this being a time in history when many people are able to have spiritual experiences and make the passageway to transpersonal levels of development. The following table published in American Health, (Greeley, 1987) illustrates polls which indicate that paranormal experiences in the USA are "on the rise."

TABLE 1:

Increases in paranormal experiences in 1973 (in parentheses) and 1986.

Americans Who:		
Had contact with the dead (adult pop.)	(27%)	42%
Had contact with the dead (widows)	(51%)	67%
Had visions	(8%)	29%

Experienced ESP	(58%)	67%
Experienced déja vu	(59%)	67%
Experienced clairvoyance	(24%)	31%
Believe in life after death	(*)	73%
Believe the afterlife is Paradise	(*)	68%
Believe that after death they'll be reunited with dead loved ones	(*)	74%

(*) No figures available

National surveys by the Gallup Organization bolster Greeley's polls showing paranormal experiences in the United States are on the rise:

Had an unusual spiritual experience	43%	('85)
Had a near-death experience	15%	('81)
Believe in life on other planets	46%	('81)
Believe in life after death	71%	('81)
Believe in reincarnation	23%	('81)
Believe in God or a Universal Spirit	95%	('81)
Believe Jesus is God	70%	('83)
Believe in angels	67% of teenagers	('86)
Believe in heaven**	71%	('80)
Believe in hell	53%	('80)
Expect the afterlife to be boring	5%	('81)

** Of those who believe, 20% think their chances
   of going to heaven are excellent.

Spiritual Experience

Although spiritual emergence, by the foregoing definition, is that process of moving into the highest levels of development, the Subtle, Causal and Atman;

experiences indigenous to these levels can occur at any time in the normal life cycle of development. These experiences have been called 'peak experiences' (Maslow, 1964, 1971), 'religious experiences' (James, 1902), 'Near Death Experience' (Ring,1984), 'transpersonal experiences' (Armstrong, 1985), 'paranormal experiences' (Greeley, 1987), conversion experiences' (Allison, 1968) and 'ecstatic states' (Eliade, 1964). When they have come as a result of drugs, either recreational or pharmaceutical, they have been more loosely termed "altered states of consciousness" (Silverman, 1971). For the purposes of this manual, we will use the term 'spiritual experience' to refer to all those experiences of the Subtle, Causal and Atman levels, which happen for any number of reasons at any time of life.

> *(spirit)...is constantly striving for release from its entrapment in routine or conventional mental structures...if this work of releasing spirit becomes imperative but is not undertaken voluntarily with knowledge of the goal and with considerable effort, then the psyche is apt to take over and overwhelm the conscious personality with its own powerful processes.*
>
> *(Perry, 1986, p.33-34)*

In spiritual experience, a person in a lower level of development is given a glimpse of a higher transpersonal level. Examples of spiritual experience are:

1. A child has clairvoyant perceptions.

2. A neurotic woman who has not yet reached mature ego functioning has an experience of

the Virgin Mary for a short period of time in
church after several nights of insomnia.

3. An 18 year-old man, lonely, depressed, and
    disoriented in his first semester at college,
    has an experience of the Low-Causal
    dissolving into God. This is not related to
    drugs.

4. A 21 year old woman living in a meditation
    community, meditating 5 hours a day, has an
    experience of the High-Causal' formlessness,
    the "suchness" of the universe.

5. A 35 year old woman, attending a breathwork
    session, has tremors of energy shaking her
    hands for 20 minutes. She later reports
    realizing she has the ability to give people
    "healing energy" through her hands.

6. A man, aged 27, writes:

    *"I have on a number of occasions felt that I had
    enjoyed a period of intimate communion with the
    divine.   These meetings came unasked and
    unexpected, and seemed to consist merely in the
    temporary obliteration of the conventionalities
    which usually surround and cover my life...Once
    it was when from the summit of a high mountain
    I looked over a gashed and corrugated landscape
    extending to a long convex of ocean that ascended
    to the horizon, and again from the same point
    when I could see nothing beneath me but a*

boundless expanse of white cloud, on the blown surface of which a few high peaks, including the one I was on, seemed plunging about as if they were dragging their anchors. What I felt on these occasions was a temporary loss of my identity, accompanied by an illumination which revealed to me a deeper significance than I had been wont to attach to life. It is in this that I find my justification for saying that I have enjoyed communication with God. Of course the absence of such a being as this would be chaos. I cannot conceive of life without its presence."

(cited in W. James, 1901, p.71-2)

Spiritual Emergency

As spiritual emergence unfolds into new areas, it can bring with it elements of surprise about the nature of oneself and one's world. This is true whether someone is actually moving to a higher developmental level, or integrating a spiritual experience into a developmental level which has not yet attained mature ego functioning. The disorientation and instability that results from intense spiritual experiences in either case, can turn a spiritual experience into a spiritual emergency. The phenomena of the crisis may last anywhere from minutes to weeks.

The capacity to integrate spiritual experiences into one's self-concept and functioning in the world is the key determinant in the outcome of spiritual crisis. A spiritual experience is more likely to turn into a spiritual emergency when:

21

1. Someone has no conceptual framework to support the experience, with which to understand and accept the phenomenon with equanimity.

2. Someone has neither the physical nor emotional flexibility to integrate the experiences into life.

3. The family, friends, and/or helping professionals of a person having the experience see the phenomenon in terms of psychopathological symptoms which have no possibility of being positive.

The pressure people place on persons in the midst of an intense spiritual experience to perceive themselves as crazy is often one of the most influential elements turning an emergence process into an emergency. Conversely, the willingness of a helper to accept the phenomena of spiritual experience and to have faith in a positive outcome, is one of the most powerful elements in changing spiritual emergency to spiritual growth.

Examples of Spiritual Emergency

A good example of spiritual emergency is the case of Everest (Lukoff & Everest, 1986). When he was a young man in his early twenties, Everest brought himself into a transcendent state of consciousness through study and concentration. Because his psychological development was too immature to manage his state, he had to act out many of the themes of his inner process at inappropriate times much to the bewilderment of his family and friends. He told them, in the midst of his intense experience:

> *"I have been through the bowels of Hell, climbed up and out, and wandered full circles in the wilderness. I have ascended through the Portals of Heaven where I established my rebirth in the earth itself, and now have taken my rightful place in the Kingdom of Heaven. ...I hoped my friends would make a similar connection and enter into an odyssey themselves. I urged them to create their own mythic vehicles and use them as guides into an odyssey as I had done."*
>
> *(Everest and Lukoff, 1986, p.130-1)*

His father, who was a general practitioner, committed Everest to a psychiatric ward soon after Everest entered his altered state of consciousness and began to talk and act differently. This state continued for two months in the hospital, during which time he had very little interaction with the staff. He was given thorazine to inhibit the psychotic-type symptoms. Even without personal support from the hospital staff, family or friends, Everest never questioned the positive value of the experience he was having. He also was able to cultivate his transpersonal experiences through his study of symbols and rituals.

At the end of two months, when Everest left the hospital, he was totally exhausted physically, emotionally, and mentally; however, he was capable of maintaining a part time job which afforded him time to rest. Part of his exhaustion may have been a side effect of taking thorazine in the hospital. He discontinued all medication on his release.

In 1985, Everest wrote about his early experience:

> *"I have gained much from this experience. I am sorry for the worry and hurt that it may have caused my family and friends. These wounds have been slow to heal. I am deeply grateful for the great victory of my odyssey. With the dawning of a new vision of life has come a new sense of purpose. From a state of existential nausea, my soul now knows itself as part of the cosmos. Each year brings an ever increasing sense of contentment."*

> *(ibid., p.142)*

He has never been rehospitalized, has led a stable work life, and has joined a church group. He is involved with community work and maintains close relationships with his family and friends. His integration of his experience is still deepening.

Everest's story illustrates a spiritual emergency in which psychological immaturity did not allow full integration of the spiritual experience at the time it was happening. His family, friends, and doctors considered Everest's experience as mental pathology, and did not support his entering it more deeply. His own understanding of his "odyssey," however enabled him to enter it fully and reap its transformational benefits.

Another example of spiritual emergency is taken from Chamberlin (1986) who worked with a group of 15 year-old boys in a psychiatric ward at the Menninger Foundation.

> *(He) taught (them) a variety of ways of altering their consciousness as a way of exposing them to alternatives to drug use. One of these methods involved biofeedback training with the eventual focus being on theta-wave training. During the time that the focus was on the theta-wave training and immediately following it, some of the teenagers developed some out-of-the-ordinary abilities. One of them began to have precognitive experiences that he perceived as strong intuitions and he needed to discuss these, particularly to validate them. Another person's reaction was more disruptive as he began to develop healing abilities. He was initially frightened by this ability. Later, he also began to notice that his electronic equipment was malfunctioning and that people in areas in which he would go would also report malfunctioning of electronic equipment. He was given some helpful suggestions about focusing his energy, at which point the electrical disruptions stopped. It appeared that this person was developing some shamanistic abilities, which in other cultures would have been given a lot of support. He was given articles to read about shamanism, and this reading resulted in a conceptual framework that was a great deal of comfort to him. However, he felt these abilities were something he did not have the time to work*

with and so he moved away from them. By not
using them they appeared to stop.

(Chamberlin, 1986, p. 2)

Conceptual Frameworks and Supportive Contexts

The reactions of Chamberlin's adolescents illustrates the
importance of an appropriate conceptual framework
and supportive social context for persons in spiritual
emergence.

Persons in spiritual emergency are deeply influenced by
their community of friends, family and health care
workers. The mini-culture in Chamberlin's ward supported spiritual emergence in contrast to Everest's social
community. Unlike most Western cultures, some cultures,
like that in Tibet, hold a view of the world which allows
spiritual experience to be integrated into normal life.

(The Tibetan culture is built on the knowing
that)...all dharmas are dreamlike, all phenomena
are dreamlike. It's seen from the very beginning
from that perspective...Since it's seen from that
point of view, when the world actually begins to
fall apart in one's experience, it doesn't become
that much of a clash, of a contradiction...I think
what has been happening in the West is the
concretization of the world as really something
solid, a permanent thing. This has been something
that has been built on since the development of
sciences and Cartesianism, so that the (dream-like

> *quality of existence) has been "kind of kept under*
> *control so to speak." Sometimes people have these*
> *kind of (spiritual emergencies) because the real*
> *nature of existence has been so repressed, and then*
> *suddenly these energies themselves spontaneously*
> *become a little bit overwhelming.*
>
> *(Sogyal, May, 1985)*

There is no comparable perspective in Europe or North America which supports spiritual awakening as part of natural human development. Thus, most of us Westerners are afraid of spiritual phenomena. They are strange to us. We need some conceptual context to help us make sense of these phenomena so that we can be more at peace with our own and more supportive of others' spiritual awakening.

Forms of Spiritual Emergency

Many contributions to creating a transcultural conceptual framework for understanding spiritual emergence processes have been made by Stanislav and Christina Grof (1984,1986). They have identified six experiential patterns which may provoke a spiritual emergency. Although these patterns may overlap, each has certain characteristic features, or elements. A familiarity with these elements is essential for anyone working with people in spiritual emergency.

The six forms of spiritual emergency identified by the Grofs include;

1. **Awakening of the Serpent Power** (Kundalini) - A radical transformation in the individual's relationship to his or her bio-energy and openess to transpersonal levels of experience. It is accompanied by powerful sensations of heat and energy streaming up the spine, tremors, violent shaking, spasms or complex twisting movements.

2. **Shamanic Journey** - A dramatic episode of a non-ordinary state of consciousness that marks the beginning of the career of many shamans. There is an emphasis on physical suffering and encounter with death followed by rebirth and elements of ascent.

3. **Psychological Renewal through Activation of the Central Archetype** - An episode of psychological renewal marked by an inner experience of perceiving oneself as being in the middle of the world process...there is an emphasis on themes of death, afterlife, and return to the beginnings of creation.

4. **Psychic Opening** - An episode characterized by striking accumulation of instances of extrasensory perception (ESP) and other parapsychological manifestations.

5. **Emergence of a Karmic Pattern** - The individual experiences dramatic sequences that seem to be occurring in a different temporal or spatial context i.e. past life time, birth.

6. **Possession** - An episode in which the individual takes on the facial characteristics, gestures and attitudes of someone else, typically diabolical in nature.

(An article which describes these patterns in more depth is reprinted in Appendix C.)

The phenomena associated with these forms of spiritual emergency can be bizarre and terrifying for someone who experiences them without understanding. In one case, a woman in childbirth was seized by a spontaneous kundalini experience which created strong, uncontrollable vibrations throughout her body. She was frightened for her and her child's life. Her nurses and doctors offered no explanation, attempting to do what they could to make the vibrations stop. For 10 years after the experience she was afraid to talk or think about the experience until finally she read about it and understood what it was. Sympathetic and knowledgeable support at the birth could have helped her enjoy the extraordinary joy that comes with the rise of kundalini.

Hundreds of stories from people who have had spiritual emergencies and have been misdiagnosed as mentally disturbed were collected by Ring (1984) and the Grofs (manuscript in process). One woman suffered through treatment for a psychotic episode after she had a mystical experience at the birth of one of her children. She had been doing hatha yoga for a year, but because her yoga teacher did not emphasize the possibility that the yoga postures might catalyze a spiritual awakening, she did not connect the yoga to her spiritual experience during the birth. In the midst of the delivery, she spontaneously perceived lights which put her in a state of awe so profound that she lost touch with her surroundings. Believed to be mentally unstable and incapable of caring for her child, she was given medication to suppress the symptoms of her supposed psychosis and directed not to breastfeed the child while she was medicated. No one had the knowledge to suggest that she may have been blessed with an experience of the Divine or had attained a level of understanding which was not only valid, but which gave her extraordinary resources as a human and as a mother.

Many types of experiences involving a spiritual awakening have resulted in humiliation and been invalidated rather than celebrated. Because our Western culture generally does not accept spiritual emergence phenomena as the product of a sane mind, most of the people who have had near death experiences (NDE) are inhibited from talking about their experiences for fear of being considered and treated as crazy.

According to Ring, people who have NDE are usually counseled by their doctors, nurses, and clergymen to forget the memories of the experience...as if it was only a hallucination or a bad dream attributable to stress. Many NDErs who have not had people to validate their experience wonder if they were crazy. Some, however, spend their lives affirming the truth of their experience in spite of their communities lack of support.

Ring wrote about one woman who met a divine being during a near death experience. Later during the birth of her child she experienced a "surge of great joy" when she realized that her child would be able to go with the divine being she met when she was in her NDE. After her baby died a few days after birth, she did not experience the grief her doctor and minister expected her to go through. She wrote:

> *"Well, I soon realized that my acceptance back into this world depended upon 'pretending' to forget, and 'pretending' to grieve the loss of my baby. So, I did this for everybody else's sake—except my husband, who believed me, and gained some comfort from it, second-hand. It was a dropped 'subject', but never forgotten."*
>
> *(Ring, 1984, p. 81)*

Clearly a change in the attitudes of the public in general and health-care professionals in particular toward the validity of NDE phenomena might produce dramatic benefits. We might not fear death, might believe in the existence of divine beings, and might feel we could talk about paranormal phenomenon.

Some of the phenomena of spiritual emergence have been misconstrued as indicators of pathology. For instance, some criteria for the diagnosis of psychosis (DSM-III, 1980) are observable in spiritual emergency:

31

1. A disorientation which makes a person less interested in work, in social contacts and in self care.

2. A difficulty in communicating about one's experience to others [in spiritual emergency this is the result of the noetic quality of the experience, not symptomatic of confused thinking].

3. Dissociation [in spiritual emergency this dissociation is a product of an attempt to integrate one's experience].

These phenomena subside after a spiritual emergency whereas in a chronic psychosis they do not. Determining whether a person is in spiritual emergency or victim of a mental disorder will be the subject of chapter 3, Diagnosis.

Summary

Spiritual emergence is a personal realization of a reality beyond ego reality, and, ultimately, one's unity with all things. The outcome of a spiritual experience may be spiritual emergence or spiritual emergency. If during a spiritual emergency the individual is given an appropiate conceptual framework and community support, spiritual emergence is made more likely.

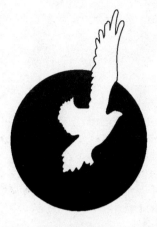

Chapter Two ─────────────────

When Does Spiritual Experience Happen?

Spiritual experience is more likely at specific times and under particular circumstances. These circumstances may be personal (as discussed in this chapter) or global (discussed in chapter 8). At the personal level, there are spiritual practices and psychopharmaceutical techniques that can serve as catalysts for spiritual experience and spiritual emergence. In addition, times of physical or emotional distress can provide the conditions for a spiritual experience to occur. This chapter includes discussion of the following personal circumstances that are often associated with spiritual experience:

I. **Time of Life:**
   1. Dark Night
   2. Destiny Calls

II. **Spiritual Practice:**
   1. Intensive Practice

III. **Physical Distress:**
   1. Athletes and Yogis
   2. Near-Death Experience
   3. Surgery
   4. Pregnancy and Childbirth

IV. **Emotional Distress:**
   1. Emotional Intensity
   2. Fragmentation
   3. Emotional Deprivation

V. **Intense Sexual Experience**

VI. **Substance Use / Abuse**
   1. Depressants
   2. Stimulants
   3. Barbiturates
   4. Opiates
   5. Marijuana
   6. Empathogens
   7. Psychedelics

Time of Life

Spiritual experiences can happen at anytime and in anyplace. A person can have an occurrence of extra-sensory perception. Very common is 'deja-vu', a sense of having been somewhere or known someone before. Also common is the knowing who is calling on the phone before the phone rings. People often experience a sense of total rightness in the world that sometimes comes as if by 'grace'. These spiritual experiences are windows into the extraordinary and may include psychokinesis, psi phenomena, occult knowledge, or mystical experience. They happen to infants, young children, adolescents, and adults of all ages without regard to time, place, or circumstance.

The Dark Night

Although spiritual experience can happen at all ages, mid-life is a time that often precipitates spiritual awakenings, particularly among individuals who have achieved some real level of stability, even prosperity in the world.

> *"They've got it, to put it in the vernacular, they've got the two kids, they've got the two cars in the garage, they've got a house in the suburbs, or whatever the New Age equivalents of those things are. They've come to some level of personal ego (development). There's a self-sense, a definition of self that's relatively well-established. Then it still*

doesn't work. Life still doesn't work. These very subtle, elusive feelings of emptiness begin to emerge, feelings of,"So What? What have I done this for?" As one of my clients put it so eloquently, using the Lennon and McCartney song,"Nowhere Man, ... I have become a real 'Nowhere Man'. " There is a yearning for something more, but not knowing exactly what it is. It's certainly not something more tangible. It's certainly not something more material. It's something more enigmatic, something that's immaterial. It's my belief that what's happening in this kind of a crisis is that the Soul/Spirit is asking, demanding to be recognized on some very deep level. That may not be what the client presents. In fact, most of the time it's not, but my experience is that as we unwind and go further into the material that the client presents, it's very very often a yearning for the Spirit, for a greater sense of wholeness that includes an abiding, eternal principle."

(Wittine, May 1985)

This experience is a modern aspect of the Dark Night of the Soul, that is, the existential encounter with meaninglessness which meets any man or woman who has reached material goals and has still not found inner satisfaction. This is the Dark Night of the Ego where life is no longer satisfying just pursuing ego gratification (Vaughan, 1985). Gopi Krishna pointed out that such an experience may also occur to an adolescent, not only the more typical mid-lifer.

> *...at a certain critical state in the development of
> the human mind the unanswered "Riddle of Life"
> attains an urgency which no treasure of the earth
> can counteract. This is the state of mind of
> millions of disillusioned young people of the world
> today...when thrwarted in its mission, the impulse
> can lead to social and political unrest...craving for
> drugs, promiscuity or other social evils and even
> to violence.*
>
> *(Gopi Krishna, 1975)*

The longing for something more may precipitate a search
for or spontaneous experience of Subtle or Causal level
phenomena. If this longing is not met satisfactorily, the
effects may be disastrous for the individual and have a
negative impact on society. The following passage
illustrates this:

> *...about 30 Americans under 21 years of age commit
> suicide every day, indicating a three-fold increase
> in the rate of suicide among American youth over
> the past decade. Also more than half the patients
> admitted to mental hospitals in the United States
> are young people...the main cause of the increase
> in the number of suicides and mental disorders
> among the youth is the increasing hollowness and
> senselessness of life of the society and the younger
> generation's distaste for profit.*
>
> *(Treffert, personal quote to Gopi Krishna, 1975)*

Destiny Calls

People who do not experience the Dark Night may instead be 'grabbed by the eternal' (Kennett Roshi, Fall,1982) through a dramatic dream, a chance meeting with an inspiring person, a drug experience, or a spontaneous awakening. These experiences impel people to advance their developmental process into transpersonal levels. This is particularly true with adolescents and young adults who are looking for a meaning to their life.

Anne Armstrong's story illustrates the autonomous quality of spiritual experience when it almost forces itself on one, regardless of one's openness to it. Anne was a young wife and mother, a Girl Scout leader, living an ordinary life in a very normal suburb. She was not the least bit interested in psychic phenomena, yet, she spontaneously began to experience psi phenomenon that would not cease. She began to meditate and undergo hypnotherapy, cultivating her relationship to these spontaneous psychic happenings. Whenever she would stop these practices, she was saddled with migraine headaches. From her perspective, the Subtle realm forced itself on Anne, as if it was her destiny to develop and become a psychic counselor (Armstrong, 1986).

Spiritual Practice

It is commonly believed that most people have entered transpersonal levels of consciousness by means of an

38

intent to grow spiritually coupled with an intense
dedication to spiritual discipline. Religious traditions of
the Far East and ancient cultures have significantly
influenced how people learn how to reach transpersonal
levels of consciousness. Lesser known esoteric Christian
texts offer this same knowledge. However, Hindu and
Buddhist literature, among others, offers a language for
transpersonal states of consciousness which is far more
detailed than anything we have in the English language
(Wilber, 1980). Practitioners of both Eastern and Western
religious disciplines are capable of reaching transpersonal
levels and equally face the difficulty arising coming from
intense spiritual practice.

Intensive Practice

Intensive practice of prayer, meditation or devotional
work in both Eastern and Western religious practice can
catalyze spiritual emergency. Following is Baraz's (1985)
description of the types of difficulty arising from intensive
meditation, and the corresponding psychological stress
that can catalyze spiritual emergency processes.

> *One meditation teacher calls practice "one insult
> after another." You see all the stuff that's in there.
> So it takes a lot of kindness and compassion with
> what you see and patience with the process. You
> see what's there and perhaps you have an image of
> what you'd like to be like. You know, a spiritual
> person who's loving and kind; and you see rage
> and fear and whatever, sadness, and that
> discrepancy can be very discouraging. That's*

where patience and compassion and kindness are essential. That's where it's very helpful to have someone around to check in with when you start getting lost in your despair. So that's the first level of difficulty that can happen.

The second one is that you start seeing that you're not who you think you are. The connection that you have with your identity, especially the good stuff, starts to dissolve. At times it can be nice when you see," Oh, I'm not the garbage" but [what follows is] "Gee, if I'm not the garbage then I'm not the good stuff, and then WHO AM I?" That can be unnerving. It's like the rug being pulled out from underneath you. As that idea of self starts to dissolve, it can get very terrifying actually.

The interesting thing is that the other side of seeing that you're not who you think you are is freedom. When you see that you don't have to hold onto anything and be so caught-up in protecting and getting recognized and all these things, there's a tremendous letting go of stuff that allows you to really have connection, on a much deeper level, with other beings...

Another thing that often happens on retreat is that concentration can open up tremendous amounts of energy. That can be very terrifying. The system starts getting, seemingly, overloaded.

I remember one retreat, the first 3 month retreat I had. After doing the [meditation practice] for a

*couple of years I did a 3 month retreat. I started to
feel like I was going to explode, literally explode.
Just bursting...like I was a sun, about to explode.
I didn't know where it was going to go and I got
very frightened. Tears were running down my
face and I went running up to the teacher and said;
"Hey, I'm just watching my breath and all this
stuff is going on. What's going on here?"*

*He said, "Oh, don't worry about it, just do this and
do this ... and breath and a few different things."*

*It was awhile before I started seeing that you can
become comfortable with that energy so that you
can become a vessel for it. If you can soften around
it and be quite still and not anticipate the next
thing, you open up your capacities to new levels of
energy. But it can be quite fearful and
overwhelming. In that state, if the mind trips out
onto a thought of "What's next?" or "I don't
know what's going on" you lose your center and
it's difficult...*

*In addition to opening up to the energy, there's all
sorts of psychic stuff that seems to happen at times,
synchronistically. You start to experience things
in a different reality than typically. Generally, if
you report those things, the teacher says;*

*"OK. Just notice them and let them go and keep on
sitting."*

41

> *[What he means is]...It's not to get stuck in having any experience, it's just to watch it all coming and going.*
>
> (Baraz, October, 1985)

Leaving an intensive retreat also can be difficult because one needs to integrate newly discovered sensitivities into a life which is far more stressful and demanding than the quiet, supportive environment of the retreat.

> *After you've left that situation where you're wide open, where you have expanded to some extent, or to a large extent, coming back into the world is not so easy, especially the first few times you do it. That transition is really important. If you think of it in terms of...an energy system that's expansive ...like a wide-open baby and this tender baby steps out on the highway and things are whizzing by...It can be jarring, to say the least. That sensory overload can be difficult to handle. The world is very fast. Your boundaries between yourself and the world are not as in place as they normally are....*
>
> *I've gotten quite a few phone calls when people have left retreats, often from another particular style of practice where there's alot of emphasis on body opening up and not much on transition. People have called up and said, "I'm having all these flashes and I don't know what to do."*

> *Also, sometimes someone is stuck in a place where*
> *everything is dissolving and it still goes on after*
> *the retreat. Although it might be a very advanced*
> *space, it's still not very pleasant. Sometimes*
> *people don't even know what's going on.*

> *(Baraz, October, 1985)*

In this final quote Baraz provided an example of a spiritual teacher helping someone deal with psychic phenomena accompanying spiritual practice. One benefit of spiritual communities is that there is likely to be a teacher or priest who can provide guidance and support if a spiritual experience occurs during intense meditation or prayer.

The attitudes of the spiritual teachers / priests (and other community members in a church or community situation) have a broad impact on how a spiritual aspirant manages a spiritual experience. Teachers, gurus, and priests differ, however, in their capacity to deal with spiritual crisis. Some are able to defuse a crisis situation; but others have little understanding of or skill in dealing with the needs of someone in spiritual emergency.

Baraz gave suggestions for helping persons doing intensive spiritual practice so that their spiritual experiences do not take them into a state of crisis. He advocated compassionate understanding and a non-judgmental attitude toward the mental confusion and emotional upset that accompany spiritual emergence. This has been the attitude of Buddhist teachers in the East as well.

43

Unfortunately, not all teachers, gurus, priests, or spiritual community members have such an attitude or the skills to work with disturbed people. Steindl-Rast made this point about monastic communities:

> *The communities in monasteries are made up of run-of-the-mill people from that particular culture. They share all the prejudices that other people in their culture share. So even though, on one level, they know...they have come to a place for spiritual emergence, and that is their path, they may also share, on another level that is closer to their reflective consciousness, all sorts of prejudice, even against mental diseases ...*

> *(Steindl-Rast, May, 1985)*

Even though the purpose of a monastic community is to support spiritual emergence, the members of the community do not necessarily teach skills in dealing with spiritual emergency (especially when emergency looks like mental disease). In their ignorance, these communities may unfortunately contribute to the disorientation and fear which can turn a spiritual experience into a spiritual emergency.

People's spiritual emergence may be overwhelming on a physical or emotional level. Offering a person a stable center, a grounding in the body and emotions, may be one of the most powerful contributions to spiritual emergence that monastic communities can offer their members (Steindl-Rast, May, 1985).

It seems to me that monasteries can and I think
actually do perform a real function in this respect,
precisely by what is often looked at negatively:
namely the many people that leave, you see? I've
always taken a very positive view of that and said,
"why worry about it?" ...I think they may be the
ones who get as much out of it as the ones that stay!
There's nothing wrong with it in many cases.
Some people find nothing. Others find what they
need, then leave. Still others stay, because they
keep finding what they need. Those who find what
they need, grow by the monastic experience. And
that's what counts, whether or not they leave or
stay.

(ibid.)

Different spiritual communities have different resources
for helping their members through a spiritual emergency.
Some communities have the capacity for supporting
their members (for example, Naropa in Boulder, Colorado), however, other communities refer their members
to psychiatrists and doctors, expecting them to handle
any emotional and physical disturbances. Chapter 5,
On-going Support, presents suggestions for helping
people who need support in spiritual emergency.

Physical Distress

Whether it be through an intensive physical workout,
disease or injury, or giving birth, physical distress is one
of the most provocative catalysts of spiritual experiences.

45

These experiences push one to one's limits of physical endurance and bring one face to face with the boundaries of life and death. This is fertile ground for the occurrence of spiritual experience.

Athletes and Yogis

The practice of hatha yoga is reputed for its ability to help people become flexible and relaxed. When practiced intensively, hatha yoga is a way of purifying the body and precipitating spiritual emergence. In intensive practice, the yogi or yogini is constantly aware of pushing right to the limit of potential—to stretch, to remain balanced, and to retain concentration. To enhance their abilities, dedicated practitioners will also restrict themselves to a very simple diet and limit their sexual activities. The result of this regimen is a high-level wellness, where yogis of any age feel full of buoyant energy, at peace with themselves and the world, and consistently growing toward the Subtle and Causal levels of their own development.

Athletes who are aerobically fit, and who push the levels of their physical endurance, also report experiences of ecstasy when they push through to a new level of energy, a second wind...or when they complete a race in which they have gone "full out." These athletes, like the yogis, have usually led very disciplined lives, restricting their sexual activities and limiting their diet, so as to stay in shape.

A serious young runner named Jim Colvin has formulated it for himself: " To run to me means to practice a religion that reflects life in a microcosm, that cleanses the entire man- mind and body- - and that allows an almost mystical communication with nature and meditation on existence...Running allows me to communicate with an inner being. ...The successful runner achieves something of the transcendentalist's solitary status in which observation and imagination blend to span the schism between mind and matter. He extends himself toward something beyond common scrutiny, something almost indecipherable, something at once natural and cultivated. A contemporary psychiatrist, Alan McGlashan, has noted in <u>The Savage and Beautiful Country:</u> "For the profoundest questions the seeker himself is the essential instrument of the seeker." The runner, in the sensual euphoria of his inner soliloquy, discovers McGlashan's "central point within oneself: the secret threshhold where the world of the senses and the world of the psyche meet in mutual simultaneous recognition." For such a moment of illumination-the eternal 'now' of the transcendentalist-dichotomies such as mental-physical, inner-outer and pain-pleasure are suspended while "a man for a timeless moment discovers his own Center." The runner often wonders whether or not he has brushed against, however momentarily, the shadow of a fourth dimension.

(Cusack, 1974, p. 23-24)

Yogis have a body of literature and a community of fellow practitioners who accept spiritual emergence to help them integrate the unusual experiences borne out of intensive yoga practice. Athletes who have spiritual experiences might well ascribe them to good health, self-discipline, or concentration, and might never think about them in the context of spiritual emergence. No matter, both athletes and yogis reap the benefits of spiritual emergence in the above cases.

Near Death Experience

Near Death Experience (NDE) refers to the experience a person has when he has been clinically dead a short period of time and been revived. It appears that NDE often introduces people to Subtle and Causal states of consciousness (Ring, 1984). It is not unusual for persons who have almost died to experience themselves as distinct from their bodies and to become aware of beings of higher intelligence and good will who are guiding them.

The personality shifts that result from NDE typically follow a pattern, which may be described as follows:

1. Confirmation in the presence of God.
2. A sense of being a part of God.
3. An unusual ability to heal and demonstrate psychic abilities.
4. A sense of deep peace.
5. A desire to be of service to humankind.

(Ring, 1984)

These are the same kinds of shifts in personality which happen to people reaching transpersonal levels of development. They especially parallel what has been recorded about kundalini awakening:

> *However the actual process of kundalini arousal may be experienced, it is held that the energy it draws upon has the capacity to catapult the individual into a higher state of consciousness. In full awakenings, a state of cosmic consciousness can be attained and, under certain circumstances, maintained. The flow of energy is said to transform the nervous system and the brain to enable them to operate at an entirely new and higher level of functioning. Metaphorically speaking, kundalini appears to throw the nervous system into overdrive, activating its latent potentials and permitting the individual to experience the world and perform in it in an extraordinary fashion...*

> *In full kundalini awakenings, what is experienced is significantly similar to what many NDErs report from their experiences. And more than that: The aftereffects of these deep kundalini awakenings seem to lead to individual transformations and personal world views essentially indistinguishable from those found in NDErs. That these obvious parallels exist does not, of course, prove that they stem from a common cause, but it does at least suggest the possibility that there may be a general biological process that underlies them both-as well as transcendental experiences at large.*
> *(Ring, 1985, p. 230-231)*

49

Surgery

Many people undergoing surgery have experiences similar to a near death experience as a result of their anesthetics (Rogo, 1984). The anesthetic ketamine seems especially effective for inducing spiritual experience. The aftereffects of the anesthetic leave patients transformed in their thinking about death, life after death, and the nature of their life.

Following is the account of a doctor undergoing surgery, having been anesthetized with ketamine:

> *He reported he heard odd buzzing sounds in his ears. He fell unconscious, but then "gradually I realized my mind existed and I could think, I had no consciousness of existing in a body; I was mind suspended in space." The doctor then found himself floating in a void. "I was not afraid," he reported, "I was more curious." He thought, "This is death. I am a soul, and I am going to wherever I should go."*
>
> *(Johnstone, 1973, p. 460-1)*

Reportedly, only 12% of those who are given ketamine in medical settings experience phenomena similar to NDE (Rogo, op.cit). Still it is a noticeable number.

Pregnancy and Childbirth

Pregnancy and birthing are especially stressful physical events which can also precipitate intense spiritual experiences and possible spiritual emergency. Miscarriage and abortion may have a similar powerful effect.

During pregnancy, birth and in the first few weeks of post-natal life, the spiritual energies surrounding a mother and child are especially intense. Clairvoyants have reported seeing beings of light surrounding the mother and child during this phase of life (Lievegoed, 1962). The hormonal changes during pregnancy, birth and lactation also bring psychological shifts which alter consciousness. Changes in sleep patterns and lack of dreaming time which accompany pregnancy and caring for an infant can also bring openings into Subtle level experiences.

The sensitive attunement mothers have for their newborn children often expresses itself through a spontaneous knowing about the welfare of the child. Women awake in the middle of the night with the inner knowledge that the child will soon need to be fed- - even when they are not keeping to a schedule other than the child's . Some women, without any outward signs, develop an uncanny knowing of when their child is in danger. These are psychic phenomena, manifestations of the Subtle level of development.

Birthing is an experience in which many women feel they are close to death, or that they have extraordinary experiences of spiritual energies protecting them and guiding them. Sometimes women have peak experiences of merging into "God's Light" while delivering a child. This can come either from a near-death experience while delivering a child, or from the exhiliration of a normal birth.

Abortion and miscarriage can also precipitate major awakening experiences—either through a confrontation with death (because of a physical emergency such as hemorraging), or a confrontation with the child's death. Even a moral crisis can precipitate spiritual experience. A woman client was struggling with the dilemma of having an "unwanted" pregnancy. As she reflected on the situation, she realized that the child was functioning in her as a spiritual awakener—helping to bring forth in her new spiritual energies for which she had always longed. She also realized that it was appropriate for her to terminate the pregnancy. Her husband agreed. After that time she continued to have expanded perceptual abilities and stronger healing capacities—all characteristic of Subtle level phenomena. She has continued to function well in her home and work life.

> *The child is potential future...the "child" paves the way for a future change of personality. In the individuation process it anticipates the figure that comes from the synthesis of conscious and unconscious elements in the personality. It is therefore a symbol which unites the opposites; a mediator; a bringer of healing; that is, one who makes whole.*
>
> *(C.G. Jung, 1968, p.164)*

Emotional Distress

Emotional Intensity

The moral choices, emotional adjustments, and life transitions associated with pregnancy, death, illness, or separation (from loved ones or loved jobs) are emotionally intense situations which often stimulate spiritual experiences. Intensive individual or group therapy produces emotional stress that can contribute to spiritual development. All of these experiences lead to confrontations about one's belief in God, a sense of what is real, and a sense of what is meaningful in life. During emotionally stressful situations, the power to create and destroy life, and the power to pull ourselves toward or away from loving relationships and creative expression, are more evident. We are also forced to acknowledge our vulnerability.

When we are vulnerable, psychological complexes that have been in the unconscious are more likely to rise to consciousness. Where there is an intense aversion to the complex, it's birth to consciousness may provoke an overwhelming reaction (Sandner and Beebe, in Stein, 1984) - thereby catalyzing a spiritual emergency.

When emotional stress is most intense there is a turning point where a person **reorients** life toward continued growth, **retrenches** in the same life patterns and self-structure, or **regresses**. The inspiration to open to continued growth most frequently comes from a personal epiphany, a spiritual experience, or a deep sharing with another person—a deepening of love, of trust, and

53

openness to life. This is most apt to happen when a helper, therapist, teacher, or compassionate friend is present.

Without the deep connection to a supportive source— personal or transpersonal—one who is in intense emotional distress typically feels isolated and overwhelmed. One may regress to lower levels of functioning, or rigidify one's identification with one's current level of development. In both cases, one is inhibiting transpersonal development.

Fragmentation

We live in a time when people feel fragmented (Metzner, May,1985) - pushed by so many economic, personal, and social stressors that no stable sense of meaning or purpose exists. Many live isolated both from their own inner core and from other people. This fragmented state is reflected in hard rock music, where there is an overwhelming cacaphony of sound that has no harmonic core.

The fragmentation is brought on, in part, by the breakdown of social institutions, and the speed at which people move from situation to situation - on the freeway, in elevators, in the air, in re-locating to different communities. A sense of continuity with others and a sense of support from one's community are unlikely.

Emotional distress induced by the lifestyles we lead and the cultural mandates which we uphold may precipitate spiritual experience and spiritual emergency.

Emotional Deprivation

Under the stress of emotional deprivation some people fall to pieces, but others grow stronger. An example is the strong child in an alcoholic family who develops psychic abilities to survive the unpredictable and unsupportive nature of an alcoholic parent. Similarly, an individual on a vision quest - fasting from food, water and human contact--can envision true purpose in life, and realize the oneness of all life. Both the child and the individual move into Subtle level experience - the one to survive, the other to intentionally stimulate spiritual growth. Each experiences deprivation and hardship, new insight and revelation.

Deprivation from human contact under circumstances where one is in emotional distress, creates a void from which can come a major spiritual awakening. When borne out of an unstable, unpredictable life circumstance, however, deprivation from emotional support can be the stimulus to emotional paralysis and disease.

Intense Sexual Experience

Intense closeness with another person can also be a powerful trigger to transpersonal development. There are spiritual practices (such as Tantric sexual practices) that are done intentionally to stimulate spiritual experience. A person in sexual activity may have Subtle, Causal and Atman level experience such as: clairvoyantly seeing the partner's past or knowing the partner's

55

thoughts; clairsentiently feeling what the partner is feeling; becoming more sensitized to subtle energies; having visionary experiences activating the "central archetype" (Perry, 1974); feeling merged with the Divine; and feeling divine inspiration.

The sexual embrace models the archetype of divine union—where male and female energies are united; where those who are separate are one and there is the experience of wholeness. No wonder that our spiritual development can be stimulated by sexual union with a beloved.

Substance Use/Abuse

Aldous Huxley (1931) was one of the most public spokespersons for drug-induced spiritual experience.

> *The story of drug-taking constitutes one of the most curious and also, it seems to me, one of the most significant chapters in the natural history of human beings. Everywhere and at all times, men and women have sought, and duly found, the means of taking a holiday from the reality of their generally dull and often acutely unpleasant existence. A holiday out of space, out of time, in the eternity of sleep or ecstasy, in the heaven or the limbo of visionary phantasy. Anywhere, anywhere out of the world.*

Drug-taking, it is significant, plays an important part in almost every primitive religion. The Persians and, before them, the Greeks and probably the ancient Hindus used alcohol to produce religious ecstasy; the Mexicans procured the beatific vision by eating a poisonous cactus; a toadstool filled the Shamans of Siberia with enthusiasm and endowed them with the gift of tongues. And so on. The devotional exercises of the later mystics are all designed to produce the drug's miraculous effects by purely psychological means. How many of the current ideas of eternity, of heaven, or supernatural states are ultimately derived from the experiences of drug-takers?

Primitive man explored the pharmaceutical avenues of escape from the world with a truly astonishing thoroughness. Our ancestors left almost no natural stimulant, or hallucinant, or stupefacient, undiscovered. Necessity is the mother of invention; primitive man, like his civilized descendent, felt so urgent a need to escape occasionally from reality, that the invention of drugs was fairly forced upon him.

All existing drugs are treacherous and harmful. The heaven into which they usher their victims soon turns into a hell of sickness and moral degradation. They kill, first the soul, then, in a few years, the body. What is the remedy? "Prohibition," answer all contemporary governments in chorus. But the results of prohibition are not encouraging.

57

> *Men and women feel such an urgent need to take*
> *occasional holidays from reality, that they will do*
> *almost anything to procure the means of escape.*
> *The only justification for prohibition would be*
> *success; but it is not and, in the nature of things,*
> *cannot be successful. The way to prevent people*
> *from drinking too much alcohol, or becoming*
> *addicts to morphine or cocaine, is to give them an*
> *efficient but wholesome substitute for these*
> *delicious and (in the presently imperfect world)*
> *necessary poisons. The man who invents such a*
> *substance will be counted among the greatest*
> *benefactors of suffering humanity.*
>
> *(A. Huxley, 1931)*

Mind altering substances have long been one answer to human yearning for a more transcendent reality. For many people, drugs have been the initiator into the Subtle realms of experience, igniting their interest in further personal development. For others, drugs have been the initiator, as well, into the hell of addiction and moral degradation.

Which drugs facilitate spiritual emergence? Which drugs facilitate recovery from spiritual crisis? Which drugs block integration of spiritual experience? The May 1985 SEN conference participants spent some time considering the effects of mind-altering substances (not including psychiatric or allopathic drugs) vis-a-vis spiritual emergence.

58

It appears that some drugs may legitimately be used to facilitate spiritual emergence **when used in the appropriate set and setting**. However, more discussion and research is called for on this subject. There is still much to be learned about this field of substance use and abuse in relationship to spiritual growth. The following paragraphs give a brief synopsis of the discussion of the 1985 SEN conference. They are included here for purposes of reflection and to stimulate further research. They are not intended as an endorsement of drug use to stimulate spiritual experience. Any experimental use of mind-altering substances must be managed with utmost care and respect for the current legal regulations as well as the psychological well being of the client. Helpers in a position of assisting persons who have used mind-altering substances may find the following review useful.

Depressants- Alcohol
This group of mind-altering substances rarely triggers a spiritual emergence of any magnitude. Small amounts of alcohol can help " turn-off " the rational mind, and thus create an avenue of expression for more inhibited emotions, thoughts, feelings and sensations. People attracted to the use of alcohol may be looking for spiritual experiences. Spiritual issues may arise out of a drying out period after too much alcohol has been consumed, but the alcohol itself does not stimulate spiritual emergence or the integrating of spiritual experiences.

Stimulants- Caffeine, Amphetamines, Chocolate, and Cocaine

These will not trigger spiritual emergence, nor facilitate integration of paranormal experiences. Stimulants, in fact, appear to block the integration of spiritual experiences. Amphetamines can, in some circumstances, precipitate psychotic episodes which may have spiritual aspects; however, they are not recommended for such a purpose.

Barbiturates

These have an effect very similar to alcohol vi-a-vis spiritual emergence. They do not catalyze spiritual experiences nor do they facilitate integration of spiritual experience. They are used, in some cases, for therapeutic purposes when sedation is important for a period of time.

Opiates- Heroine, Morphine, and Opium

Opiates can stimulate Subtle level experiences in some people. The opiates stimulate imagination and fantasies, which can lead to out-of-body experiences and visions. When used wisely, opiates can help people in pain so that their minds are free to deal with spiritual issues and can thus help integrate spiritual experiences in special circumstances.

Marijuana

Marijuana is in a class between the opiates and psychedelics. It can produce new sensory experience, initiate a person to spiritual experience, and help integrate spiritual experiences. Its capacity to do this depends on the intent of the user, the dosage, the quality, the set and the setting.

Empathogens- MDMA (aka Adam, or Ecstasy)
This is a drug that can open people to spiritual experience. It often awakens the heart center, opening people to the here and now. It facilitates the integration of spiritual experience if used in the appropriate dosage and setting. Side effects are generally minimal and short-lived.

Psychedelics
Psychedelics can have a useful effect for promoting growth into higher levels of development when taken in the appropriate setting, with the intent for personal growth. Dosage levels must be monitored carefully, the environment must be especially peaceful, and follow-up procedures must be attended with care. Stan Grof (1980) discusses psychedelics used in a therapeutic setting.

> *The main objective of psychedelic therapy is to create optimal conditions for the subject to experience the ego death and the subsequent transcendence into the so-called psychedelic peak experience. It is an ecstatic state, characterized by the loss of boundaries between the subject and the objective world, with ensueing feelings of unity with other people, nature, the entire Universe, and God. In most instances this experience is*

61

contentless and is accompanied by visions of brilliant white or golden light, rainbow spectra or elaborate designs resembling peacock feathers. It can, however, be associated with archetypal figurative visions of deities or divine personages from various cultural frameworks. LSD subjects give various descriptions of this condition, based on their educational background and intellectual orientation. They speak about cosmic unity, unio mystica, mysterium tremendum, cosmic consciousness, union with God, Atman-Brahman union, Samadhi, satori, moksha, or the harmony of the spheres.

..In general, psychedelic therapy seems to be most effective in the treatment of alcoholics, narcotic-drug addicts, depressed patients, and individuals dying of cancer. In patients with psychoneuroses, psychosomatic disorders, and character neuroses, major therapeutic changes usually cannot be achieved without systematically working through various levels of problems in serial LSD sessions.

(Grof, 1980, p. 36-38)

The positive effects that are possible with psychedelics and empathogens are not commonly attained when drugs are taken in a recreational setting, without the intent for inner growth and without monitoring of set and setting by a trained guide. Nevertheless, it is possible for people to have spiritual experiences unintentionally through drug use - as drugs can be powerful catalysts for psychic and psychological phenomena.

Summary

Individual stressors press people toward change—to find new resources and to cope with change. Any of the stressors noted above (time of life, spiritual practice, physical distress, emotional distress, intense sexual experience, substance use/abuse) can catalyze spiritual emergence or emergency. The direction of the person's experience is often affected strongly by the Helper involved. If the Helper is cognizant of spiritual emergence phenomena, he or she can support positive change in the distressed individual. Where the Helper is ignorant of spiritual emergence processes, the distressed individual will not likely resolve the difficulty in a positive way.

The next four chapters provide information on working with persons in spiritual emergency and emergence.

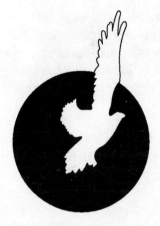

Chapter Three ───────────────────

Diagnosis

This chapter focuses on the criteria for distinguishing spiritual emergence and spiritual emergency from pathological states. Because some of the characteristic behavior patterns in spiritual emergency are similar to psychotic symptoms, it is critical to identify the differences so that an accurate diagnosis can be made. This discussion will clarify why spiritual emergency is also appropriately named an acute psychosis with a positive outcome (Dabrowski, 1964; Grof, 1985; Lukoff, 1986).

There are three ways in which people respond to spiritual experiences. One way is to integrate the experience into their lives, moving forward in their self development to the Subtle, Causal, or Atman levels. Another response is to be overwhelmed for a period of time, experiencing a spiritual emergency but eventually acknowledging and accepting the spiritual experience as a part of their reality. The third response is to fail to integrate the spiritual experience, and to deteriorate into a chronic state of confusion.

As an example of the possible responses, imagine three persons who have an experience of unity with the Divine, a Causal experience.

The first person, say a woman, is initially immersed in a greatly expanded consciousness, totally absorbed in the experience of being God and yet can flexibly shift to going on with her life - taking care of her family and the rest of life as always, doing laundry, getting children to school on time, and so on.

The second person, say a man, is so disturbed by the experience, he cannot function for several weeks. His partner assumes his household duties while he is taken care of by a support group. He needs time to rest and reflect. He feels disoriented. He can't be trusted to drive safely. His reflexes are slowed. At times, he is so energized he can't contain himself and talks on and on. He has realized he is God, and all other people are God, too. It's a big awakening. Eventually he is able to resume normal functioning, having integrated his experience into his reality.

The third person, say a woman, is initially overwhelmed by the spiritual experience, and as time goes on she grows more confused. She falls more deeply into a state of dissociation with herself. At times, she believes she alone is the second coming of Christ, or the Angel Gabriel. At other times, she is a person paralyzed with infantile fear. Her identity is constantly shifting. She lacks a stable core as a result of unsuccessful ego development. Her attention span is poor. She is difficult to talk to. It is hard for her to relate to others. She loves her children, but is so self- absorbed that she cannot attend to her needs, let alone theirs.

A classically trained psychiatrist or psychotherapist following the standard diagnostic system, DSM-III (1980), would probably categorize all three of these people as psychotic based on the **content** of their experiences.

With notable exceptions, most psychiatrists and psychologists since Freud assume that hallucinations, dramatic experiences of uncontrolled energy, paranormal phenomenon, and feelings of unbounded unity are symptoms of deep mental pathology. Visions which absorb a person's waking awareness in a dramatic play of archetypal images are similarly discounted. Psychic phenomena are invalidated because they cannot be repeated or understood by means of Newtonian-Cartesian scientific principles. Freud felt that all these behaviors and perceptual experiences were symptoms of regressive tendencies. He did not consider that they might also be part of the initiation to higher developmental levels.

Many professionals in the field of psychology often hesitate to talk about their own transpersonal experiences for fear of being considered psychotic. Their ambivalence results in their being uncomfortable discussing similar experiences of their clients. They lack understanding or interest in transpersonal experiences, and may even be willing to consider mystical experiences only within the context of religion.

Jung and Assagioli were two notable exceptions who understood that some elements of the unconscious are transpersonal in nature, are superior to ego-consciousness, and contribute to optimal well-being. Contemporary theorists and clinicians following the lead of Jung and Assagioli have reconstrued the rigidly held negative image of acute psychoses, seeing in them the possibility of a phase of disintegration which when complete would contibute to psychological well-being (Boisen, 1962; Dabrowski, 1964; Laing, 1972; Grof, 1985).

Following is a table which illustrates the diversity of opinion and vocabulary among psycholologists and psychiatrists regarding spiritual emergency.

Table 2

Name	Spiritual Emergency?	Symptom	Treatment
Freud (1924)	no	Regression and/or hallucinations: probably of organic etiology.	Medically-oriented hospitalization. Drugs.
Jung (1932)	yes	Autonomous process arising out of the unconscious that uses client as its vehicle; evidence of complex previously split off.	Jungian analysis or psychotherapy; grounding with creative work and family activities.
W. Reich (1949)	yes	Organism efforting towards unitary functioning and/or merging of organismic and cosmic orgone energy.	Vegetotherapy and character analysis; comprehension of cosmic and organismic orgone energy functions.
B. F. Skinner (1953)	no	Presence of negative conditioned response patterns.	Conditioning techniques to change behavior and interpersonal aspects of client's life.
Maslow (1971)	yes	Phenomena related to evolutionary growth.	Permission for spontaneous expression and trust in the organism.
Assagioli (1977)	yes	Crises of spiritual awakening.	Informed guide to educate client re: spiritual awakening.

Table 2: cont . . .

Name	Spiritual Emergency?	Symptom	Treatment
GAP * (1976)	no	A form of ego-regression defending against internal or external stress.	Medically oriented hospitalization; drugs, as needed, to suppress symptoms.
J. W. Perry (1974)	yes	Psychological renewal; evolutionary step.	Empathic listening, supportive, egalitarian, informed companionship; 24 hour care in home-like atmosphere.
Mindell (1984)	yes	Individuals are channels for larger process taking place in the Universe.	Process-oriented psychotherapy.
Grof (1986)	yes	Spiritual emergency.	Sympathetic and compassionate guidance from a helper; 24 hour care in home-like setting; holotropic therapy.
Lukoff (1985)	yes	Mystical experience with psychotic features. (MEPF)	Same as Perry.

* Group for the Advancement of Psychiatry

Psychosis and the DSM-III

According to the American Psychological Association's (APA) diagnostic manual of mental disorders, the DSM-III (1980), symptoms of psychosis include the following:

1. Delusions.
2. Hallucinations.
3. Incoherence or loosening of associations.
4. Markedly illogical thinking.
5. Behavior that is grossly disorganized or catatonic.

As is evident, these criteria do not differentiate the delusions and hallucinations of the psychotic from the visions and psi phenomena of spiritual experience; nor the 'word salad' characteristic of the psychotic from the jumbled speech of someone trying to articulate the noetic quality of a spiritual experience; nor between the catatonia of the psychotic with the need for solitude and quiet of the person in spiritual emergency; nor the disorganized behavior of the psychotic and the bizarre behaviors of a kundalini experience. Any of the six patterns of spiritual emergency described by the Grofs could be confused with symptoms of psychopathology as the following table suggests:

Tabel 3:   Symptoms -
Spiritual Emergency vs. Psychopathology

FORM OF SPIRITUAL   SIMILAR CRITERIA
EMERGENCY   IN <u>DSM-III</u>

FORM OF SPIRITUAL EMERGENCY	SIMILAR CRITERIA IN DSM-III
1. Kundalini Awakening: Streaming energy, tremors, sensations of heat/cold, spasms and violent shaking, involuntary laughing/ crying, unusual breathing patterns, and/or visions of light.	Autonomic hyperactivity associated with *generalized anxiety disorder* Hyperactivity associated with *manic states.* Alteration in physical function. Symptom not under voluntary control & psychological factors judged etiologically evolved- associated with *conversion hysteria.*
2. Shamanic Journey: Dreams/visions/sensing- evoking a special connection to animals and nature. Core psychic experience= death and rebirth	Recurrent thoughts of death. Loss of interest or pleasure in ritual activities associated with *depression.* Somatic, grandiose, religious, nihilistic or other delusion without persecutory or jealous content associated with *schizophrenia.*
3. Psychological Renewal Through Activation of the CentralArchetype. Preoccupation with death, rebirth, and/or return to the beginnings of life. Focus on a clash of opposites and dramatic resolution of this opposition.	Bizarre delusions. Hallucinations associated with either *schizophrenia* or *psychosis.* Recurrent thoughts of death associated with *depression.*

FORM OF SPIRITUAL EMERGENCY	SIMILAR CRITERIA IN <u>DSM-III</u>
4. Psychic Opening: Experiences of extrasensory perception, including out-of-the-body experiences.	Delusions. Hallucinations associated with *schizophrenia* or *psychosis*.
5. Emergence of a Karmic Pattern: Experiencing dramatic sequences which seem to be occurring in a different temporal - spatial context.	Delusions. Hallucinations associated with *schizophrenia* or *psychosis*.
6. Possession States: Face and/or body involuntarily take on character of another personage. Somatic consequences may include choking, vomiting, and frantic motor activity.	Symptom not under voluntary control. Loss of or alteration in physical functioning associated with *conversion hysteria*. Behavior that is grossly disorganized associated with *psychosis*. Hyperactivity associated with *manic states*.

The difficulty in making these differentiations is that the content of the visions and sensory phenomena may be identical in psychosis and spiritual emergency. Thus, differentiating pathological psychosis from spiritual emergency must be based on other criteria which enable the clinician to make finer distinctions.

Criteria for Spiritual Emergence

Such criteria for identifying a person in spiritual emergence were defined by Grof and Grof (1986).

1. *Episodes of unusual experiences that involve changes in consciousness and in perceptual, emotional, cognitive, and psychosomatic functioning, in which there is a significant transpersonal emphasis in the process, such as dramatic death and (re)birth sequences, mythological and archetypal phenomena, past incarnation memories, out-of- body experiences, incidence of synchronicities or extrasensory perception, intense energetic phenomena (Kundalini Awakening), states of mystical union, identification with cosmic consciousness.*

2. *The ability to see the condition as an inner psychological process and approach it in an internalized way; the capacity to form an adequate working relationship and maintain the spirit of cooperation. These criteria exclude people with severe paranoid states, persecutory delusions, and hallucinations, and those who consistently use the mechanism of projection, exteriorization, and acting out.*

(Grof and Grof, 1986, p. 8)

Flexibility to adapt and accommodate to new areas of experience is part and parcel of the spiritual emergence process—in contrast to inflexibility, which characterizes deeply entrenched psychosis.

Criteria for Spiritual Emergency

To determine whether a person is experiencing a spiritual emergency, two sets of criteria should be employed; criteria for a spiritual experience and criteria for a positive outcome of a psychotic episode:

> The criteria for a spiritual experience include:

1. Sense of newly-gained knowledge.
2. Perceptual alterations.
3. Delusions (if present) have themes related to mythology.
4. No conceptual disorganization (Delusional metaphorical speech which may be difficult to understand, but is comprehensible and should not be considered conceptually disorganized).

> (revised from Lukoff, 1985)

If two out of the following four criteria are satisfied, a psychotic episode is likely to have a positive outcome:

> 1. *Good pre-episode functioning as evidenced by no previous history of psychotic episodes, maintenance of a social network of friends, intimate relationships*

with members of the opposite sex (or same sex if homosexual), some success in vocation or school.

2. *Acute onset of symptoms during a period of three months or less.*

3. *Stressful precipitants to the psychotic episode such as major life changes: a death in the family, divorce, loss of job (not related to onset of symptoms), financial problems, beginning a new academic program or job. Major life passages which result in identity crises, such as transition from adolescence to adulthood, should also be considered.*

4. *Positive exploratory attitude toward the experience as meaningful, revelatory, growthful. Research has found that a positive attitude toward the psychotic process facilitates integration of the experience into the person's post-psychotic life.*

(Lukoff, 1985)

Following is a table which illustrates the determinants of spiritual emergency vis-a-vis brief reactive psychosis (a type of psychosis included in the DSM-III (1980) which is most similar to spiritual emergency, in terms of professionally used terminology, and thus most often confused with spiritual emergency).

Table 4: Psychosis or Spiritual Emergency?

BRIEF REACTIVE PSYCHOSIS	SPIRITUAL EMERGENCY
Psychotic symptoms appear immediately following a recognizable psycho-social stressor.	Phenomena usually follow a recognizable psycho-social stressor; good pre-episode functioning. (Lukoff)
Emotional turmoil and at least one of the following: 1. Incoherence or loosening of associations. 2. Delusions. 3. Hallucinations. 4. Behavior that is grossly disorganized or catatonic.	All of the following: 1. Ecstatic mood. (Lukoff) 2. Sense of newly gained knowledge. (Lukoff) 3. Perceptual alterations. (Lukoff and Grof) 4. Delusions have themes related to mythology. (Lukoff and Grof) 5. No conceptual disorganization. (Lukoff) 6. Positive, exploratory attitude toward the experience as meaningful. (Lukoff and Grof) 7. Capacity to form and maintain an adequate working relationship. (Grof)
Symptoms last more than a few hours, but less than 2 weeks.	Symptoms last minutes, and up to months; acute onset during 3 months or less. (Lukoff)
An eventual return to the premorbid level of functioning.	Functioning enhanced after most intense period is complete. (Lukoff and Grof)

BRIEF REACTIVE PSYCHOSIS	SPIRITUAL EMERGENCY
No period of increasing psychopathology preceding the psycho-social stressor.	No period of increasing psychopathology preceding the psycho-social stressor. (Lukoff and Grof).
Disturbance is not due to any other mental disorder or organic disorder.	Disturbance is not due to any other mental disorder or organic disorder. (Grof)

COEX Systems

Growth to new developmental levels almost never happens in a direct linear course. As people develop past the normal ego levels, most need to work with and resolve issues left from earlier developmental levels, such as old griefs, angers, and patterns of thinking and feeling, before emerging into a transpersonal level of functioning and experiencing.

S. Grof's (1985) 'COEX' system may be useful to describe why people regress to more primitive levels of functioning during their progression to transpersonal levels of consciousness. COEX stands for "systems of condensed experience" in the psyche. These are systems of traumatic experience at the primary level that are not fully metabolized on a primary level (such as those occurring while one is still in the womb or at birth), but which continue to exist in one's psychic structure as one matures, inhibiting full development. In order to dissipate the energy caught in the COEX system and to free the psyche a regression to the primary level for the purpose of healing is necessary. In this instance, the psyche regresses to a more primitive level in order to integrate past traumatic material. A person in spiritual emergency may, for a while, be in a more primitive and regressed state to resolve and integrate a COEX system before emerging to a higher level of integration. An episode of regression to pre-personal functioning may thus serve as a gateway to a transpersonal level of functioning. Wilber's spectrum of self development (Chapter 1) identifies the developmental levels - but not the course of development itself.

As one approaches the Subtle level dysfunctional patterns of seeing and relating to the world from preceding developmental levels will be challenged. The non linear pattern of growth explains the emotional outbursts, dramatic physical sensations, even the phenomena of "emerging of a karmic pattern" or "kundalini rising." These may be the psyche purging complexes left from previous developmental levels.

Summary

Learning how to distinguish between spiritual emergency and mental disorder is essential in providing appropriate disagnosis and care for people in spiritual emergence. Persons misdiagnosed may be caught in treatment modalities which are inappropriate and even destructive to their growth. Hospitalization for 'disease' is not appropriate and may be devastating for a person in spiritual emergency.

The specific bundle of emotions, physical sensations, and extraordinary inner states which occur in spiritual emergency come from a combination of past developmental issues and present spiritual experiences. In a person with a relatively stable ego identity, past developmental issues can be largely resolved by giving appropriate emotional support which allows the client to clear inner conflicts and accommodate the newly emerging self-structure. The next several chapters describe how to give appropriate care to a client in spiritual emergency.

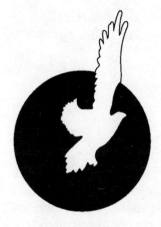

Chapter Four

Initial Interaction: Client and Helper

What occurs in the initial meetings between a Helper and someone in spiritual emergency is critical. In the initial encounter a Helper must determine whether a person is in a spiritual crisis or if he or she is experiencing a more severe psychological imbalance. This chapter explains eight steps to be used in the first interactions with a person who appears to be in spiritual emergency. They are:

1. Evaluating a medical check-up.
2. Discouraging use of psychiatric drugs.
3. Providing a quiet and safe environment.
4. Providing compassionate and knowledgeable companionship.

5. Making a diagnosis.
6. Educating the client about spiritual experience and/or emergence.
7. Helping with grounding, centering, or catharsis.
8. Referring the client.

1. Medical Check-up.

A person in spiritual emergency needs to be checked medically to determine if his or her symptoms are due to an organic imbalance. Alterations in perceptual, emotional, cognitive and somatic functioning could be caused by a gross brain disorder such as infection, tumor, cardiovascular problems or degenerative diseases of the brain. Psychological imbalance could result from physical diseases such as uremia, diabetes, toxic states, or cardiac disease (Grof, 1986).

A medical check should also determine if the person is getting adequate rest, proper nutrition, and enough liquid to prevent dehydration. During a psychological crisis of any nature, many people fail to get enough rest, and/ or adequate foods. Adequate intake of vitamins and minerals has a noticable effect on psychological health. Simply giving a person time to rest and ensuring he or she receives proper nutrition can be a potent treatment for spiritual emergency.

Adequate exercise is also important to health and psychological well-being. A sedentary lifestyle can have a profoundly negative effect on psychological well being.

2. Minimal use of Psychiatric Drugs

Psychiatric drugs should be used minimally because they tend to inhibit the natural processes which are occurring in spiritual emergency as the self-structure attempts to integrate a spiritual experience. These drugs can either slow down this natural process, or in some cases, curtail it.

Another significant reason for the minimal use of psychiatric drugs is to allow a person to be observed in his or her more natural state. This is essential for successful diagnosis. Psychiatric drugs often distort or render inaccessible a client's inner process.

3. Quiet and Safe Environment

A person in spiritual emergency is typically in a highly sensitized emotional and physical state. The person can be easily overstimulated by strong light or loud noise. Strange people such as physicians, psychiatrists, or nurses, can be very disturbing. Every caution should be taken to provide a quiet, pleasant environment.

The ideal environment for the first meeting with a client in spiritual emergency is a place with natural lighting, soothing colors, quiet music, and simple furnishings— an atmosphere that is more like a home than a hospital. Such an environment can help to allay the fears of persons in spiritual emergency and allows them to focus on their inner processes rather than on outside stimulation.

4. Compassionate and Knowledgeable Companion

A person in spiritual emergency needs the companionship of someone who truly understands this experience. Ideally, this companion will have personally experienced a spiritual emergency, or intense spiritual experiences. The companion can thereby have compassion for the client and understand the client's experience.

Ideally the companion should know about spiritual emergence processes and be able to educate the client on what is happening. The Helper is a companion and witness to the journey of the client, trying to help the client understand and integrate his or her experiences. Chapter 6, "The Role of the Helper," gives a fuller description of qualifications for a helper.

5. Diagnosis

The first interaction with a client is the time to determine if the client is in spiritual emergency. To do this, the Helper should identify the client's current psycho-social stressors and any COEX system that may be operative. (Sometimes a full diagnosis cannot be made in the first interaction.)

The Helper who is responsible for initial diagnosis needs to know about both psychological illness and spiritual emergency because of the possible confusion of spiritual emergency with other mental disorders. Fine distinctions must be assessed. For instance, borderline personality disorders can masquerade as spiritual emergency (Vaughan, May, 1985). Sometimes the confusion may be perpetrated by the client who prefers to see a disturbance in terms of spiritual emergence, which is more exciting and inspiring, than a stubborn personality disorder. Narcissistic individuals may enjoy the romance and specialness of seeing themselves involved in spiritual emergence. Hysterical personality types may be seeking permission to continue their neuroses under the guise of spiritual development, "legitimizing" the neurosis in their own and others' eyes.

The issue of diagnosis is complicated because the client may be experiencing both phenomena of spiritual emergence and symptoms of a personality disorder, organic mental disorder, or affective disorder. In such case, the diagnosis and treatment become very difficult even for the most qualified. The diagnosis and treatment may be impossible for anyone not well versed in psychological literature, professionally skilled in psychotherapy, and personally experienced in the vagaries of spiritual emergence processes. The qualifications (that is, knowledge, skill, and sensitivities) of the Helper are of utmost importance in the diagnostic phase.

Clients who are not in spiritual emergency but who have had or are having an intense spiritual experience still need help to integrate this experience. The same eight steps appropriate for conducting an initial meeting with a person in spiritual emergency are also appropriate for these clients, although they may not need as much on-going support. They need access to resources such as meditation groups, breathwork sessions, transpersonally oriented therapists, and appropriate reading materials.

6. Educating about Spiritual Emergence Process

One of the most frightening aspects of spiritual emergency is that the client (and his or her family) often doesn't know what is happening. The client may be afraid of some energy that has taken hold, or afraid of newborn psychic abilities, healing abilities, or psychokinetic phenomena. Usually, the client feels like a victim of bizarre circumstances.

A Helper must provide a conceptual framework to structure the client's understanding of spiritual experiences and spiritual emergence. This helps the client accept the emergency as positive and allays fear. Educational materials, books, articles, and movies can be introduced at appropriate times which help the client see that other people have undergone similar or identical experiences. Wilber's developmental spectrum of consciousness is a useful framework to base an explanation of spiritual development. A list of reading materials on spiritual emergence is provided in Appendix D.

Ideally, the companion or Helper can help bridge the intellectual understanding of spiritual experience gained from such resource materials with the phenomenological experience.

7. Help with Grounding, Centering and/or Catharsis

When clients first come in for help, they are usually in disoriented and disorganized psychological states. Although full of emotional and physical sensation, the clients may try to control these sensations so as not to appear crazy. They may be completely absorbed in their inner worlds, not caring to communicate with other people. They may be excited, speaking as fast as possible, jubilant and expressive or they may be profoundly depressed. Persons in spiritual emergency may appear in any number of moods.

There is no one therapeutic approach to use with a person in spiritual emergency. Grounding, centering or stimulating catharsis however, are commonly needed during the first encounter. It can be assumed that all those who come for therapeutic help are in need of some grounding. They need reassurance from others that they will be okay. They need some help to understand what is happening to them. A compassionate Helper acts as a container, holding all of the different parts of the person that are not yet integrated, and accepting the person's inner conflicts without demanding coherence. A compassionate Helper can allow the client to be a needy infant in Prepersonal consciousness one minute and a highly evolved being in Causal consciousness the next. The Helper's compassionate attitude is the most important resource needed by a person in spiritual emergency.

The clients may also need cathartic release. They need a place where it is absolutely okay to be physically out-of-control, to let go, to stop holding onto their feelings and sensations which need expression. Ideally, Helpers trained to enable cathartic release should be available at any time clients need their help. A Helper who sanctions and enables cathartic release in this way can speed the process of moving from spiritual emergency to emergence. Ideally, there would also be a safe space, cushioned and sound-proofed, for the client to do cathartic work at the appropriate times.

Spiritual emergency often manifests in very physical terms, for example, body tremors, flashes of heat, feeling healing energy in the hands, and so on. Touching the client—a hand on the shoulder, a back rub, a foot rub - may reassure the client and have a grounding effect. More sophisticated bodywork such as massage, acupressure, or breathwork is also often helpful to a client in dealing with spiritual experience on the somatic level.

Stan Grof has innovated Holotropic therapy, a group breathwork experience that helps people progress with spiritual emergence. The therapy is based on both cathartic work and grounding. Holotropic therapy is appropriate for clients in a moderate phase of spiritual emergency where they are not overstimulated, or severely underbounded, and have the capacity to contain their inner experiences with minimal external assistence.

8. Referral

After the initial diagnosis of spiritual emergency has been made, the Helper may find it appropriate to refer a client to another Helper or group for support.

In the most intense phases of spiritual emergency, a client may need 24-hour attention by sympathetic, compassionate, and knowledgeable people. Because there are at the present time only a few places in the United States which provide this service (see Appendix D), Helpers may need to design 24-hour support systems in their community outside an institutional setting. This can be especially difficult in communities or with families with little or no understanding of spiritual emergence. Intentional communities and spiritual groups that share a common desire for psycho-spiritual growth seem best suited to provide 24-hour care for their members. Often, however, even these groups are not prepared to provide 24-hour care. There are alternatives that can be employed when such care is unavailable.

Case Study

What are the alternatives to 24-hour care? I will use an experience I had as an example. Bill, an accountant, had been practicing meditation outside of any formal religious group for a number of years . He was seeing me once a week for therapy to help him loosen muscle spasms in his throat which he felt were psychosomatic in origin. I had seen him for a year when he went into spiritual emergency.

Bill was sleeping only 3-4 hours a night, talking to himself a lot, having emotional outbursts which were uncharacteristic of his former inhibited style, and seeing visions of the Virgin Mary. He remained grounded enough to drive safely and rework his schedule to accomodate more inner time. Bill himself was not frightened by the strange behaviors but his wife and family wanted to give him psychiatric medications immediately so he would "return to his old self." Bill wanted "refuge to go deeply into his experience" without the distractions of ordinary life and the fears of his family. He also wanted some companionship, perhaps "a priest, or someone who could understand the experiences he was having."

There was no place immediately available for Bill in the San Francisco Bay Area where he lived. As his Helper I did the following:

1. I made every attempt to educate the family about Bill's situation, advising them about Bill's need to have permission to go through his experience without medication. I reassured them that Bill was not crazy but was going through a very intense period of growth that would probably last a matter of days or weeks.

2. I informed Bill's wife of what she could do to help him—take him for walks so he could get fresh air and be nurtured and grounded by the beauty of nature, give him heavier foods like cheese and meat to eat, and not expect him to return to his "old self."

3. I made myself available as a support person for Bill's wife. I acknowledged the difficulty of her position, the fears she had, the strangeness of Bill's experiences and behaviors and how well she was doing in helping him. I told her to call me, or another support person, whenever she felt she or Bill needed support. I told her to call me if she noticed him being self-destructive, extremely disoriented, or fearful. I arranged for her to see a therapist at her request.

4. I kept in contact with Bill. I called him at home on the days I did not see him in my office. I asked him consistently if he was having trouble, feeling afraid or feeling self-destructive. (I was alert to possible paranoia or suicidal ideation. If Bill had been paranoid, suicidal, or a threat to anyone, I would have modified his treatment plan to include more intensive care, even hospitalization.) I reassured him that his process, however strange, was valuable and good.

When I saw Bill for our sessions in the office, I asked him how he was and listened respectfully as he recounted his experiences. During his spiritual emergency, we did not work very much with the meanings of his experiences. Grounding work was more appropriate for Bill. After a period of talking, I gave him acupressure to balance and ground his energies and to give him a physical reassurance of our connection.

5. I contacted a psychiatrist at a local hospital with
    a good reputation for working with psychotics
    using minimal medication. I informed the
    psychiatrist about Bill so that, in the event Bill had
    to be hospitalized, I knew whom to call at a
    moment's notice. I wanted to be in agreement
    with the psychiatrist who would be treating Bill
    that it would be preferable if he were not given
    any drugs in the event of hospitalization. In the
    six weeks of Bill's spiritual emergency, he was
    never hospitalized. However, my knowing that
    the backup was there was reassuring for me.

Bill could afford to take time off work during his spiritual
emergency. His wife was also in a position to come home
at lunchtime, leave work early, and take some extra days
off to be with him. Their relatively relaxed work schedules
allowed Bill time to be with himself, and gave him
meaningful and consistent contact with someone who
cared for him.

During Bill's spiritual emergency his throat spasms
disappeared. He gained understanding and clarity about
his spiritual direction. After the crisis he had a surge of
creative inspiration which he expressed through
composing, playing, and recording music. He deepened
his spiritual connection with his wife. He committed
himself more deeply to his own development (I think this
was inspired by our work together and by his reading
books I referred to him about spiritual emergence.) He
learned how to set limits with his in-laws around their
involvement in his personal life. He gained confidence

that he could manage a spiritual emergency if it happened to him again. Furthermore, Bill's wife started to become more actively involved in her own inner development.

Bill's case also affected my professional life. I was working at the Transpersonal Counseling Center at the time Bill was my client. My peer counselors offered me support and facilitated my referral to the psychiatrist at the local hospital. My supervisor, a psychiatrist, supported me in advising Bill not to take any medications. The psychiatrist at the hospital supported my assessment of Bill's situation and the concept of using no psychiatric drugs. In summation, I realized I had a network of community support and a number of Bay Area resources for helping people in spiritual emergency.

A Helper's referral network is an important resource. No single individual can be as effective in spiritual emergency as a group of persons who can provide different kinds of support 24 hours a day. Being a Helper to a person in spiritual emergency is an intensely demanding service. Thus, the Helper's support network is valuable for both the Helper and the client to process the spiritual emergency positively.

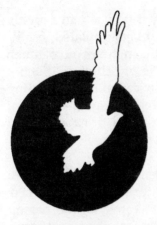

Chapter Five ───────────────

On-Going Support

Once a person in spiritual emergency has been diagnosed
and given initial assistence, it is necessary to provide on-
going support by:

1. Providing a safe environment.
2. Facilitating grounding.
3. Restructuring response patterns to increased
   energy levels ("getting unstuck").
4. Supporting spiritual emergence.

This chapter describes each of these ongoing steps in
detail.

A person in spiritual emergency is typically in a highly sensitized state - overwhelmed, overstimulated, frightened, disoriented, self-absorbed, sometimes out of touch with other people and incapable of self care. Such a person may be experiencing new capabilities - reading other people's thoughts, perceiving archetypal themes of life, seeing and palpably feeling auras, or experiencing several episodes in time simultaneously.

A person in spiritual emergency needs emotional reassurance, insight into the nature of the experience, and perhaps physical support. Above all the person needs to have someone confirm that the novel inner experiences are valid and valuable.

A person in spiritual emergency needs a particular kind of environment and a particular kind of personal help to integrate visions, insights and kinesthetic experiences into ongoing life. The person needs help to undo inhibiting emotional and physiological response patterns, to be able to contain and use expanded sensitivities, awarenesses and energy which come with spiritual experience. On-going treatment of each individual must be tailored to the person's developmental stage of growth, and the resources of the community.

Providing a Safe Environment

A safe environment is one in which the inner processes of the person can proceed without interruption and one in which the companions of the person provide support. Specifically, a safe environment includes:

1. A quiet, home-like setting with access to nature, that makes few demands on the client so that the client has the time and opportunity to explore and express his or her inner experience.

2. Companionship that supports the client's inner work and further understanding of spiritual emergence.

The Setting

Metzner (1985) reported a case in which a client was admitted to a psychiatric ward overwhelmed with constant voices in his head and unusual visions in front of his eyes which prohibited him from verbal interaction. The man was put in a small, soundproofed room where he was asked to lie down on a mattress. The lights were dimmed to almost total darkness. There was nothing else in the room except the man and the cot.

Metzner told the man that he would be on the other side of the wall and instructed the man to signal him by way of an intercom whenever the man saw visions or heard voices. To Metzner's surprise, he heard very little from his patient for 25 minutes. Finally, Metzner interrupted the man, "What are you experiencing?" His patient answered lucidly, "Finally-peace."

From this experience, and his subsequent interactions with the man on the ward, Metzner deduced that the man had such a high sensitivity to outside stimuli that he became quickly overwhelmed in an environment of bright light, noise, or people moving around. When he was emotionally supported and looked after in an environment of minimal stimulation he became centered and no longer felt victimized, frightened, or out of control. At that point he gained perspective about what was happening to him and learned to manage it.

An innovative kind of environment for people with schizophrenic symptomotology is described in an article in Appendix C of this manual. It is entitled "Soteria: An Alternative to Hospitalization for Schizophrenics." It illustrates the kind of work that has been initiated by a few psychiatrists to explore alternative therapeutic environments.

Learning how to manage one's expanding sensitivities is the most important aspect of growing into higher developmental levels. The environment that is most suitable to this task is a place of quiet, with low light, either no noise or soothing music, access to a natural setting, and access to a space safe for catharsis. An aesthetic arrangement of furniture that pleases the eye and sense of touch has a dramatic effect on subduing an overstimulated psyche.

This environment is much closer to a monastic setting that feels like a home for normal people than a psychiatric ward for sick people. But, similar to a psychiatric ward, it is an environment where a person can be totally supported physically, if need be, and reassured emotionally within a humanistic context that does not rigidly hold to the formal rules of any particular religion.

The Companions

There should be few social demands placed on a person in spiritual emergency. A demanding child or a needy friend is not an appropriate companion, whereas a supportive friend who is interested in personal development is.

Sogyal (1985) described the qualities of the interpersonal environment most appropriate for someone in spiritual emergency. He referred to the culture of Tibet:

> *People know about it (spiritual emergency) before they get it so that when it happens, generally speaking, rather than panicking, they have something to refer to, they're not alone. Actually the opening is a further clarification of what their whole education had already been illuminating for them: that the material world reflects only a small part of reality...*

> *There are cases when they do kind of freak out. Then it is the environment that helps a person through. Such an environment includes compassion, understanding, the confidence that inspires, warmth, and humor. (For the Tibetans, cultivating the quality of kindness is of uppermost importance.)*

*...for such people (in spiritual emergency)
environment is more important than anything
else, because, when you reach to that level, you
begin to have a problem relating to the environment,
to the world. So creating some kind of environment
which is stabilizing (is extremely important).
Nature is very wonderful since we are very much
related. This is the place of natural growth and
this is the place where you can grow.*

*...When these people break through, like in a death
experience and also a new birth experience, they
become like little children. The loving environment
is a very important aspect. We have to think in
terms of creating an environment for them that is
loving, understanding and stable. They also need
some basic kind of support system.*

*Environment is more important than analyzing
what is wrong or using a technique. Often we may
make mistakes in our analysis when we start
analyzing things (chuckle).*

(Sogyal, 1985)

When Anne Armstrong, now famous as a psychic
counselor, was going through her initial spiritual
awakening she was at first very frightened. She had out-
of-body experiences and past-life recalls that changed
her perspective of reality. Armstrong acknowledged the
critical importance of people who supported her and
encouraged her to explore the experiences and to trust
them.

The first time around I turned it off because I felt I couldn't cope with it, I didn't understand it, I didn't know anything about this area. I wasn't even aware that there might be a way of negotiating with this other part of myself. I felt that it was out to get me, to manipulate me. Instead it was out to give me an expanded awareness, a higher level of consciousness. The experiences were probably brought about by my meditation practice, but at that time I didn't know that. A lot of people will have a tendency to squelch it as soon as it happens, because frequently it comes in very bizarre ways. I don't really feel that it means to frighten you or to manipulate you, but we're all making so much "head noise" that it's very difficult for that part of the self to speak to us. Usually it speaks in a very gentle or a very quiet voice, but, if we don't listen to it, it may do something bizarre to get our attention.

(Armstrong, 1985)

Fourteen years later Armstrong began to work with hypnotherapy, seeking relief from migraine headaches she had had since being a young girl. Fortunately she was at a time in her life where she could take 2-3 hours a day for therapy and meditation. Anne's husband became an active partner in her process and worked with her using hypnotherapy to help her find a way to understand her evolution into higher consciousness. Armstrong wrote that it was the loving acceptance others gave to her, and her study of diverse religious texts which helped her integrate her extraordinary experiences.

Through hypnosis I found the way into that opening again. The second time around, thank God, I was a little more knowledgable...I felt in control, which I feel was the major difference between the first time I had the opening, and fourteen years later. The second time, I felt totally in charge. I felt that no matter what happened, there was some part of me that in some sense was 'minding the store', and that I didn't have to worry about it. There needs to be some way to communicate this to a client who is having spontaneous out-of-body experiences, hallucinations and other related phenomenon, as I was. They need to be assured that there is a part of the self, that I call the Witness or the Monitor, that is always "on guard," that is always looking out for your best interests. Once you learn to trust this Monitor, you lose the feeling of being a victim. So I went from feeling victimized by the energy to saying, "What is this energy and what can I do with it?" I made friends with it.

Also, another thing that was very helpful was that I had a therapist who understood exactly what was happening to me. Fortunately the universe brought these kinds of people in to me. And I also had a very supportive husband, who was fascinated by the process. So, instead of saying "You're crazy!" he'd say, "Now, what's going on? What else can we do with this new tool that we have?" Fortunately, I was in very good hands. And I feel that it's very important for the therapist to understand that there can be spontaneous emergence of these other levels of consciousness,

*that it can manifest as past life recall, as
hallucinations, and various kinds of paranoid
feelings and actions. The therapist needs to be
supportive, no matter what the client comes up
with. My therapist and my husband treated my
fears and past life recall as if they were real.
Whether or not they were real is irrelevant. The
important thing is that that part of my self was
being given expression and I was getting more and
more trust in myself and my process. So let me say
it again, <u>the supportive environment was very
important</u> (author underlined.)*

(Armstrong, 1985)

Facilitating Grounding

*To be grounded is another way of saying that a
person has his feet on the ground. It can also be
extended to mean that a person knows where he
stands and therefore that he knows who he is.
Being grounded, a person has "standing", that is,
he is "somebody." In a broader sense grounding
represents an individual's contact with the basic
realities of his existence. He (or she) is rooted in the
earth, identified with his body, aware of his
sexuality, and oriented toward pleasure. These
qualities are lacking in the person who is "up in the
air" or in his head instead of in his feet.*

(Lowen and Lowen, 1977, p.13)

Paradoxically, spiritual experiences often take people outside the context of their religious affiliation. It is difficult or impossible to find words or scriptures that adequately describe the experience. A spiritual experience is totally unique, and at the same time universal— connecting one to all of life. One of the most liberating and, at the same time, frightening qualities of these experiences is that they are beyond words, beyond normal reality and normal expression.

An important strategy for integrating transpersonal experience is to 'ground' oneself, that is, to come back to earth and to oneself after being in a 'space' that seems "out of this world." The following list of techniques can be helpful to ground clients when they are "spaced out" and feel disconnected to people and the physical world. It is also important to teach clients in spiritual emergence how to ground themselves, and to recognize when they need grounding.

1. Stay in contact.
2. Stay in the present moment.
3. Affirm boundaries.
4. Support creative expression.
5. Affirm connection to people and nature.
6. Eat grounding foods.
7. Do simple rhythmic activity.
8. Do grounding visualizations.
9. Read books on spiritual emergence.
10. Minimize the use of psychiatric drugs.
11. Create meaningful rituals.

1. Stay in Contact

Be available to talk to persons in spiritual emergency in a way that is engaging. Maintain eye contact. Touch them by giving them light (non-sexual) massage. Affirm their experience by putting it in a positive framework. Be trustworthy.

2. Stay in the Present Moment

Ask the clients to tell you what sensations they are having in their bodies. Ask them to tell you what they perceive in the room in a concrete way, for example, "I see the plants in the corner. They have long, droopy leaves about 2 feet long. They are next to the door that is painted blue. The rug is beige. There are 10 pillows lined up against the wall." This helps people orient to their surroundings and differentiate who they are from what is around them. This is especially useful when a person is feeling frightened by a unitary experience or is underbounded for other reasons.

Share emotions and your bond to the client. For example, "I love you, I want to be with you as long as I can, I feel honored you are sharing your experience with me." Do not relate emotions that can be interpreted as divisive. For example, "I hope that never happens to me." Ask the persons to tell you what they want. For example, "I want to eat some pudding...I want to have a back rub...I want you to hold my hand and not talk."

3. Affirming Boundaries

All people have a strong sense of personal space around their bodies with which they identify. Persons in spiritual emergency may be highly sensitive to other people entering their personal space. Affirm that you are aware of their personal space and you do not want to violate that space by forcing intimacy or support on them.

Kathlyn Hendricks (1985), a dance therapist, suggests asking persons to identify their personal space by pressing against the imaginary line of their boundaries with their hands. Doing this all around the body can give them a stronger sense of their own identity and help them communicate to another person how they experience their personal space.

Resting and bathing can also help them ground and identify with their own sense of space.

4. Creative Expression

Supporting persons to express the nature of their spiritual experiences through expressive dance, artwork, sandtray, clay, music, or poetry also helps them find a means to communicate to others and reconnect with their world. Artistic expression is a language of symbol and metaphor which can help clients bridge the spiritual experience with ordinary consciousness. Gay Hendricks (1985), a body therapist and clinical psychologist, tells people to "give it away. Experience all of what is happening to you—then give it away." How one can share one's emotional response to a spiritual experience might be through a hug, a dance, or any other creative expression.

5. Affirm Connection to People and the Natural World

When a person in spiritual emergency has difficulty relating to other people, a walk in nature can provide a stabilizing source of connection to the earth and the physical world. Just taking a walk in an area where there are trees and growing things is a powerful reminder of the earthy simplicity of life, that each thing that grows has its own individual pattern of growth. Pets can also provide a grounding experience.

Grounding can be greatly facilitated by connecting to a few people or a group who are all involved with spiritual emergence. It is especially important that all in the group identify with their own development to transpersonal levels and thereby affirm their own and others' experiences. All forms of sharing can also help ground— holding hands, singing, chanting, telling one's story, or a creative expression of one's spiritual experience. Groups engender a sense of belonging and provide a context where one is seen for one's extraordinariness, as well as accepted for one's part in the larger whole.

Stanislav and Christina Grof ask people in their groups to draw mandalas depicting their experience after experiential therapy. Each person is then given the opportunity to show his or her work to the group. The picture itself communicates something of the nature of their experiences often more clearly than the person's verbal description. Gathering in a circle to share experiences of this nature is preferable to gathering in a way where people cannot see each other's faces. The circle includes everyone as equals. Each person faces the group. No one person stands out as leader, or authority, or outsider.

6. Grounding Foods

What we choose to eat has a lot to do with how we feel. A light diet of mainly fruits, vegetables and grains can help people to stay slim and feel light. Vegetarianism may help people to attune to the more subtle energies of life, which are the gateways and guideposts of the Subtle and Causal realms. Denser foods such as meat and dairy products have the effect of helping people identify more with the grosser energies of the physical world. The denser foods are more difficult to digest and therefore demand more vital energies in the process of digestion and assimilation.

A person in spiritual emergency may benefit by a diet heavier in meat and dairy products as it will help bring the person down to earth. On the other hand, if a person is in a spiritual emergency coping with unpredictable rushes of energy, the person's system may be too imbalanced to be able to handle much, or any, food at all. There are many differing opinions about diet and it is not within the scope of this handbook to cover diet in any depth. Certainly, when a person is in crisis the body is usually in a highly sensitized state and will benefit from a simple diet devoid of food additives and preservatives. Fresh air is also a boon to anyone in this state.

7. Simple Rhythmic Activity

Walking, housecleaning, baking bread, sweeping the floor, raking leaves, weeding, swimming, and other easy-paced activities which have some repetitive rythmic movement in which the whole body comes into coordinated motion are all excellent for grounding.

8. Grounding Visualizations

Persons in spiritual emergency are identified more with the world of extraordinary phenomena than with the earth and its relatively slow rythms. Visualizations can be used to foster a reconnecting with the earth. Ask these persons to feel their feet on the ground, to feel the support of the earth underneath them, or to imagine a line going from the base of their spine and anchoring to a spot in the core of the earth. The shorter and simpler the instruction the better because persons in crisis will often not have long attention spans. They may also be suffering from feeling lost in their own inner world, and a visualization which takes them further into their own inner world could be negative.

It may be wise for persons who meditate to decrease the amount of time they spend in meditation while they are experiencing a spiritual crisis. It may be better for them to stop meditating altogether for a time, rather than amplifing the inner world drama by continued meditation. This decision must be made on an individual basis because some meditations can serve as powerful grounding devices whereas others are designed to upset persons from their habitual grounding.

9. Books to Read

Books about people who have experienced spiritual emergence/emergency in a positive way provide models for people attempting to make sense out of their own disturbing spiritual experiences. Reading about someone else's experience can be very reassuring, and often inspiring. In Appendix 'D' is a list of reading material useful to anyone wanting to understand the phenomenon of spiritual emergence.

10.   Minimize Psychiatric Drugs

Most psychiatric drugs inhibit the process of spiritual emergence by preventing potentially therapeutic catharsis, dulling inner awareness and unbalancing the body's own homeostatic process. The side effects of many psychiatric drugs take energy away from the process of moving into a higher level of awareness or from the process of grounding. Some psychiatric drugs increase disorientation, and inhibit personal contact that is so crucial to a person in spiritual emergency.

One of the participants at the SEN conference (1985) had been institutionalized because he could not carry out his duties in the military. At the time he was very involved in his inner process. In the psychiatric hospital he was given phenothiazine and thorazine. He described these drugs as "debilitating, and (preventing him) from staying present with what was happening." He inferred they interfered with his journey of awakening to higher levels of self development.

In Appendix C is a report of a study on people hospitalized for schizophrenia who were treated without phenothiazines. The results indicated that some schizophrenics have a better chance of recovery when left to work through their processes in a non-drugged state.

Some institutions have established settings for people in psychological crises where psychiatric drugs are not preferred treatment (Telles, Perry and Price, 1985). Diabysis was an institution for the care of first-break psychotics in San Francisco. A ward of Agnews State Hospital in California also functioned for a time with minimized drug use. Both of these treatment facilities attempted to provide safe environments and both reported positive outcomes from their clientele. Unfortunately both facilities folded for lack of funding, even though the cost of treatment per client was less than in traditional facilities and fewer clients were reinstitutionalized.

11. Ritual

Ritual focuses attention and can be particularly useful with people who are distracted or overwhelmed and are trying to regain a sense of stability.

Universally, ceremony and ritual have been used to evoke elevated feeling and to remind people of the presence of spiritual forces. As people develop towards the Subtle level they become more palpably aware of the presence of universal energies. Participating in ceremony which formalizes reception of higher wisdom can help persons who are overwhelmed by spiritual emergency.

Some of the common rituals are ceremonial dance, listening to music, watching a fire or candlelight, spiritual singing and chanting, prayer and meditation. Community participation accentuates the power of any ritual, although a private ceremony done alone or with a few people can also serve well to focus spiritual energies.

The grounding effect of ritual is that it gives definition to energies that are not visible and are seemingly out-of-control and unpredictable. The symbols used in religious rituals represent spiritual energies in visible form. For example, the blood of Christ is imagined in the communion wine. When we drink the wine, we symbolically take in the spirit of Christ. Tibetan Buddhist Thangkas (religious paintings) are symbolic renditions of the energies of God, which are used in meditations to evoke higher spiritual energies in the meditator.

Creating a place which is sacred and used for ritual only can be very important for grounding. A corner of the living room for a small altar and book of prayer can provide a sacred place in one's home to stimulate one's awareness of spiritual energies. Religious objects can also be used as a focus. Giving a person in spiritual emergency a religious object, for example, a crucifix for a Catholic, or a small statue of Kuan Yin for a Chinese Buddhist, can be especially helpful.

Assisting those in spiritual emergency to find a religious ceremony or symbol that has particular meaning for them and to which they can create a lively bond is a powerful way to help. Formal religious ceremony has usually served this role, however, there are more and more people who develop their spiritual awareness outside of any religious institutions.

It may be appropriate for a Helper to introduce a symbol from a different culture that can enhance spiritual understanding for those in spiritual emergency. For example, the Hindus have a goddess called Kali who embodies very different energies than any feminine religious symbol known in the West. Kali is an awesome creature with a necklace of skulls adorning her neck, her tongue dangling out of her mouth, her eyes bulging out of her head, and her long black hair blowing wildly. She symbolizes the energies of chaos, death and change. She affirms that change is part of life, that ignorance dies and wisdom is born in change. Knowing Kali as a religious symbol can assist a person undergoing spiritual emergency to recognize the value of chaos and change as an opportunity to grow into higher realms of knowledge.

Ritual and symbol create boundaries and structure for unbounded and unstructured experience. They are a way to integrate spiritual experience with worldly experience, and to focus on growth toward higher levels of development.

Getting Unstuck

Letting go of old emotional patterns and physical tensions which limit range of movement and growth is part of the process of spiritual emergency. A helper must be able to facilitate clients' changing response patterns, help them to intensify their connection with their inner process, and help expand their awareness of their new level of consciousness. Establishing therapeutic rapport, trans-personal breathwork and energy balancing are three techniques that are especially useful in helping clients in crisis to make these changes. Each demands some training, but does not require a graduate degree.

Establishing Therapeutic Rapport

The full attention of a Helper who is both empathic and respectful of the inner experience of an individual in spiritual emergency is a powerful healing force. It encourages the individual to give significance to his or her own inner process. Furthermore, the intensified awareness of the inner process helps these individuals process the emotional response to their spiritual experience.

> *This 'therapeutic' rapport with another seems to*
> *provide a containing framework for the individual,*
> *within which the process can be experienced in its*
> *fullest intensity and yet in some measure of*
> *security. It does not seem particularly important*
> *that the person in the 'therapist' position be able to*
> *make 'interpretations' according to any*
> *psychological theory; an empathetic participation*
> *with the Individual in the inner experience seems*
> *to be sufficient.*
>
> *(Perry, 1974, p. 153-154)*

Thus, empathic participation helps clients to be fully in their inner process.

The Helper does not need to have any special training to be able to give full attention to individuals in spiritual emergency. Simply employing principles of active listening (Speeth, 1982; Young, 1983) is sufficient. However, a Helper may need to have experienced altered states of consciousness many times in order to be present with the client without being worried or feeling pressure to make the client conform to expectations of normalcy (Perry, 1974).

There is little need to interpret and analyze the clients' inner experience until the spiritual crisis is over and the clients are in the process of integrating the experience. At that time, helping clients interpret the experience is a vital part of the therapeutic process.

Establishing rapport with clients involves forming a relationship which has some depth of intimacy. The

Helper must function as a close friend and guide, caring, giving without expectation of return, respectful of the inner life of the client, providing safety, and yet simultaneously, allowing the clients' full experience and expression of their inner process.

Transpersonal Breathwork

Transpersonal breathwork is a natural physical and psychic stimulant useful when clients need a catalyst for self-expression. As breathwork raises energy in all systems of the body, it increases the possibility of breaking through inhibiting response patterns to increased levels of energy. Results range from spiritual experiences, to remembering forgotten important life events, to deep energetic or emotional experiences, to learning how to manage higher levels of energetic expression.

Breathwork is not advised for people who are at a stage in their spiritual emergence when they are overstimulated and need grounding. It is also contraindicated for pregnant women and people who are recently out of surgery, or have a heart condition or epilepsy.

It is advised for people in phases of spiritual emergence when they are relatively grounded and need to be more closely aligned with their emotional and bio-energetic life. Jacquelyn Small (1985) finds breathwork highly effective with drug addicts and alcoholics in recovery. It is also very effective in training Helpers because it can lead to experiences of altered states of consciousness.

People in spiritual emergency usually dissociate to some degree, separating from their emotional response to their spiritual experience. This happens because they have not yet learned how to contain or manage the larger amounts of energy that come with spiritual experience. Thus, they need special help to connect fully to their inner process and learn new patterns of response to heightened energy levels, to express and contain rather than repress or dissociate. This connecting reduces their fear of what is happening to them, because it gives them the feeling of being at one with themselves. This helps clients trust the process of spiritual emergence as positive.

Doing breathwork stimulates the body's own homeostatic processes. If persons need to let go chaotically in order to come into balance within themselves - the breathwork will move them closer to a chaotic letting go. If persons need to have visions to assist them in their evolution, they will be likely to have a vision. If persons need deep peace, they will be likely to have that experience. Personal volition, desire from the ego, and the voluntary nervous system are less influential during breathwork than the autonomic nervous system—which is in charge of homeostatic processes both in the body and mind.

"Breathers" may have any number of inner experiences during a session. Chronic muscular tension becomes more apparent and may heighten and then spontaneously release. Emotional catharsis can also occur. The release of muscular tension may stimulate insight into emotional complexes and COEX systems. "Breathers" may review physical trauma, feeling and expressing the emotions that were not expressed at the time of the trauma. They

117

may experience enlivening energy streaming in their bodies and they may have visions or Subtle sense perceptions characteristic of transpersonal states.

Transpersonal breathwork should always take place in an environment which is private, protected, and supportive. In a breathwork session, the therapist allows anything to happen excepting sexual acts and actions that could hurt someone. The breathers are encouraged to trust their inner knowing, surrender to what is deeply felt, and to stay in touch with their own inner process. A significant aspect of this work is that it provides a social context which supports this way of being. The context in the breathwork demonstrates to people that there is a place in life where it is appropriate to totally let go, to connect fully with inner process, to express fully, to surrender to the unknown.

At the end of breathwork sessions, which last 1-2 hours, participants in a group are asked to gather together and share their experiences. Similarly, in an individual session, a breather reports to the therapist and thus, grounds his or her experience, verbally reinforcing the learning and gaining objectivity.

Breathwork comes out of the shamanic and ancient yogic traditions, which use breathing techniques and evocative music to catalyze spiritual experiences, and from Reichian therapy, which uses breathing techniques and deep tissue massage to catalyze emotional catharsis and psychological integration.

Breathwork has been criticized as a mystification of hyperventilation because people often feel dizzy and / or get muscular spasms around their mouths, hands and feet which are characteristic of hyperventilation. It is now, however, well established by breathwork therapists (Cucuruto,1977; Jackson, 1984; Hendricks and Hendricks, 1985; Grof, 1985) who have seen thousands of people in hundreds of sessions, that dizziness and muscular spasms subside as a person accommodates to higher levels of energy in the body. Dizziness and spasms appear to be linked to chronic patterns of muscular tension that interfere with natural energetic flow and muscular holding - characteristic of people who are holding down their energetic capacities.

I believe it is important for people to have individualized attention from a trained breathwork therapist during most of their breathwork sessions. By doing specific body manipulations the trained therapist will assist the breather in re-educating his or her body to find a new pattern of containing high energy and expressing it in an integrated way—a way in which the body maintains alignment and balance, and the person knows when it is appropriate to express and when to contain expression. Without individualized assistence, breathers will still break into areas of themselves that have been repressed because of the increased energy charge of the breathwork activity itself and they will have the characteristic experience of peacefulness after the session, but, they will not necessarily retrain themselves to manage increased energy smoothly.

Training to facilitate breathwork with an individual or a group is important. Breathwork can stimulate powerful experiences on any level—physical, emotional, or spiritual. A Helper facilitating breathwork needs to have a strong background in being both a 'breather' and a 'sitter', a companion to the one who is breathing. 'Sitting' with anyone in deep emotional states like rage, grief, fear, and love can train Helpers to stay centered in high stress situations such as spiritual emergency. A breathwork facilitator also needs training in how to release energy blocks which are painful and sometimes occur in a session, for example muscular spasms in the throat or chest which inhibit breathing, severe tension in the shoulders, or cramping in the stomach or legs. The breathwork facilitator must also educate the clients about what to expect from breathwork and how to manage the phenomena which arise both during and after the session. The facilitator also needs to be skilled in identifying when people are dissociating and in helping them become grounded.

Energy Balancing

Evolution has a biological basis, and every transition in human development has its somatic expression. Infants are enabled to differentiate from their parents as young children when they gain the capacity to walk out of sight of their parents. Young people are enabled to differentiate more fully from their families when they make sexual bonds with a mate and establish their own families. The bridge between the higher egoic levels and the Subtle realms is possible when a person can consciously use large amounts of energy in a balanced way.

> *All the systems of Yoga and all religious disciplines are designed to bring about those psychosomatic changes in the body which are essential for the metamorphosis of consciousness. A new center—presently dormant in the average man and woman—has to be activated, and a more powerful stream of psychic energy must rise into the head from the base of the spine to enable human consciousness to transcend the normal limits. This is the final phase of the present evolutionary impulse in man. The cerebrospinal system of man has to undergo a radical change, enabling consciousness to attain a dimension which transcends the limits of the highest intellect. Here, reason yields to intuition and revelation appears to guide the steps of humankind.*
>
> (Gopi Krishna, in White, 1984)

The energy system of a person in spiritual emergency needs to be considered when the Helper is creating a treatment plan. Bodywork designed to align and balance a person with his or her natural flow of energy is helpful in spiritual crisis. Examples of energy balancing techniques include accupressure, acupuncture, Lomi, and Rosen work. These forms of bodywork are less active and more structured than transpersonal breathwork. They are advisable for people in spiritual emergency who are too ungrounded for breathwork or in a vulnerable physical condition.

121

SEN maintains a referral system and can assist people who want transpersonal breathwork or energy balancing to find an appropriate Helper trained in these modalities.

Supporting Spiritual Emergence

After a client has had a spiritual emergency, how does a Helper assist the client's subsequent growth? This section explores three basic elements necessary to support development into Subtle and Causal levels:

1. Maintain a positive attitude
2. Identify a map of the journey
3. Invite new ways of being

Maintain a Positive Attitude

Maintaining a positive attitude toward development into Subtle and Causal levels is an essential support to a client's growth. Such development can be a difficult process because it requires that we disidentify with our familiar ego state and explore unknown perceptions and awarenesses. The journey into new realms can be frightening, just as it can be ecstatic.

Buddhists believe that the mainstay of support in the journey of transpersonal development is "taking refuge in the Triple Gem." The Triple Gem refers to Buddha, Dharma and Sangha.

To take refuge in the Buddha means acknowledging the seed of enlightenment that is within ourselves, the possibility of freedom. It also means taking refuge in those qualities which the Buddha embodies, qualities like fearlessness, wisdom, love and compassion. Taking refuge in the Dharma means taking refuge in the law, in the way things are; it is acknowledging our surrender to the truth, allowing the Dharma to unfold within us. Taking refuge in the Sangha means taking support in the community, in all of us helping one another towards enlightenment and freedom.

(Goldstein, 1976, p.1)

This Buddhist wisdom applies to anyone in any religion. It is a universal truth that the seeds of our highest potential are within us. We need only to nourish those seeds and be with people who support us.

Finding a community of friends who will support one's process of spiritual emergence is a blessing. Such friends can be people inside or outside of an institutionalized religion who recognize that human growth proceeds past ego development to levels of wisdom, compassion, and creativity which are extraordinary. The friends might be a group who meet to meditate together, or to discuss writing about the transpersonal realms.

All people who value the states of mind associated with transpersonal realms and want to experience them, and there are many, can be considered supportive friends for someone in spiritual emergence. Many groups have evolved to support their members within a group context. The most consistent support for self development will come from the group with whom one shares the most in common—a similar meditation practice, a common living place, or the same spiritual guide.

Physical places can serve to support one's spiritual emergence. A church, the birthplace of a spiritual leader, a mountain retreat , a ritual mound built on top of a lei line are all places which serve to stabilize and inspire one in the intention to grow to higher levels.

Support for spiritual development can also be received from things, animate or inanimate, which reflect to us our deepest nature. This may be a figure from our dream lives, a person who comes to us in meditation, a flower, a candle flame, a child, a dog, anything that serves to guide our own unfolding.

Some people who have progressed into transpersonal levels of development believe they have communicated with and felt support from the spirits of people who have passed away. Da Free John communicated with Shakti (the Divine Cosmic and Manifesting Energy) and the spirit of his dead teacher, Swami Nityananda .

> *Then, one day, to his great surprise and immense good humor, the Shakti manifested Itself to him in visible form as the Virgin Mary. She began to guide his spiritual practice. Eventually, she told him to go on a pilgrimage of the major Christian holy places in Jerusalem and Europe. Master Da related these experiences to Bhagawan Nityananda,*

who appeared to him in a vision. Nityananda told him that he belonged to the Mother Shakti now and that She (The Divine Spirit-Presence, In Person) would be his Guru or Guide. With Nityananda's Blessings, Master Da left India to carry out the Mother's instructions. In the course of his pilgrimage, Master Da was released of his remaining emotional ties to Christianity. Indeed, he was released from the total past, and he emerged simply in Love with his "Blessed Companion."

(Da Free John, 1985, p.33)

Identifying a Map of the Journey

Maps of the journey to the Subtle, Causal and Atman realms of development can be found in three places: one's inner psyche, a teacher (or teachers) who models the way, and books which literally map the path and give instructions for specific spiritual practices.

One's own inner psyche often points the way through dreams or visions. Jung's story of his life in <u>Memories, Dreams and Reflections</u> (1961) is an example of this. Jung was not drawn to the Eastern way of working with a spiritual teacher and also felt alienated from his father's church and the religious institutions of his community. It was through his dreams and inner reflections that Jung became aware of his longing for the experience of the Divine. This led him into a journey of intensive study, research, writing and retreat, where he went more and more deeply into his experiences of the Divine.

Sometimes psychic pressure produces a vision which becomes a beacon and guides us towards transpersonal reality. According to Bolen (1984) the heroine in classic folk stories (meaning the woman who will discover the transpersonal truths and bring them back to society) frequently feels alienated from her family as a child, feeling that her parents are not her real parents. She develops a vision of meeting her 'real family' later on in life after she has accomplished some of the necessary tasks of her own growth. The 'real family' is the group who will acknowledge her higher transpersonal self, relating to her with deep love, compassion, and wisdom. This vision then inspires the girl to live with patience, perseverence, and to maintain her awareness of higher reality.

The map of the journey can come from a spiritual teacher who models the path to higher development by his or her own lifestyle, inner attainment, and teachings. In this context, a spiritual teacher is anyone who has attained the Subtle, Causal or Atman levels of development. This person is then in a position to teach other people about spiritual emergence by sharing experiences of his or her own journey and teaching them techniques used to catalyze transpersonal growth.

Spiritual teachers have not necessarily qualified themselves to teach through a particular course of study, or a specific discipline aimed at self-development. Many people who have experienced the Subtle and Causal realms (for example, through a Near-Death Experience) have the ability to transmit their wisdom. These people are spiritual teachers because they have the ability to transmit the quality of the experience and thus be guides to some extent.

The ideal spiritual teacher has integrated his or her own spiritual experiences, and who is geographically nearby, perhaps a yoga teacher, a meditation teacher, a member of the Native American Church, a minister or priest. Each serves to support growth toward transpersonal levels of self-development. The best spiritual teacher has attained transpersonal levels of development. How does one recognize a person who has reached the highest level of development?

> *In the traditions of yoga certain guidelines are given to help distinguish one who is advanced from one who isn't. In the Bhagavad Gita, Arjuna asks his teacher how can one identify a man who is firmly established and absorbed in the highest consciousness. He is told that such a person is "not shaken by adversity," that he is " free from fear, free from anger" (Bhagavad Gita, Ch.2). The way the teacher sits is carefully scrutinized. He who is restless with poor posture betrays his lack of control over the body and reveals a dissipated, unfocused mind. The way he walks is observed; whether it indicated hurriedness, a sense of being torn and pressured, a posture of defensiveness, or whether, on the other hand, it reflects confidence, ease and self control. Speech is also evaluated. Is one distracted, wandering, rambling, losing the thread of the conversation? Is he critical and negative in his comments about others? Does he tend to focus on the negative aspects of everything*

127

*around him, and do his own actions tend toward
destructiveness? Does he become angry for no
apparent reason, misinterpreting what others say
and do, distorting them so that they fit his own
ideas?*

*One need not ask the customary question about
hallucinations, bizarre ideas, etc. to distinguish
such a person from the mystic who despite his
"strange ideas" presents a vastly different picture.
The traditional observations amount to a prag-
matic sort of descriptive psychiatry. The authentic
mystic reflects an inner discipline - despite the fact
that his ideas and behavior may be difficult to
understand. However baffling his speech or actions,
he nevertheless reflects an inner peace-through a
relaxed body and harmonious coordination, and
through patience, confidence, clear thinking and
an unselfish attention to the needs of others.*

(Rama et al., 1976, p. 205-206)

The support of such a person helps point the way to inner
peace, compassion, and energetic creativity.

Many types of literature can serve to guide one in spiritual
emergence. Personal accounts, ancient texts and
scriptures, or instruction books on how to perform specific
exercises all give a map of the journey. The Autobiography
of a Yogi (1946), the story of Yogananda, an East Indian
who came to the United States to teach about Yogic
principles as well as Christian philosophy, is one of the
most widely read stories of personal evolution.

Poetry, music, and various art forms including architecture and dance can also serve to evoke in people a feeling for higher levels of consciousness. The ecstatic poetry of Kabir, a 15th century Indian influenced by the Sufis and Hindus, spoke directly of the inner knowledge which comes in the Subtle level:

> *Are you looking for me? I am in the next seat.*
> *My shoulder is against yours.*
> *You will not find me in stupas, not in Indian shrine rooms,*
> *nor in synagogues, nor in cathedrals:*
> *not in masses, nor kirtans, not in legs winding around*
> *your own neck, nor in eating nothing but vegetables.*
> *When you really look for me, you will see me*
> *instantly-*
> *you will find me in the tiniest house of time.*
> *Kabir says: Student, tell me, what is God?*
> *He is the breath inside the breath.*
>
> *(translated by Bly,1971)*

Judith Whitman-Small's contemporary poetry is similarly inspiring:

> *The sacred space expands*
> *in all directions*
> *making the whole world*
> *an altar for worship.*
> *Light the incense of devotion*
> *to all life*
> *and watch its healing smoke*
> *spiral past*
> *the boundaries of the mind.*
>
> *(Small, 1985)*

129

These two poems point to the experience of God, to that which is sacred outside the limitations of a specific religion. They point to an experience that may be found anywhere, by anyone.

Most of the literature we have pertaining to higher levels of consciousness is contained in particular religious writings, which seems to imply that the higher states are accessible only to people who follow a particular religious path. In fact, the higher states of consciousness are available to anyone, inside or outside of a formal religious setting. Literature which illumines this is liberating for people seeking spiritual development.

Inviting New Ways of Being

Spiritual teachings and transpersonal therapies are designed to evoke new ways of being which are less centered on egoic consciousness and more attuned to transpersonal consciousness. The individual who wants to grow into these higher levels must seek out the teachings and therapies appropriate for himself or herself.

Shirley MacLaine began to explore transpersonal realms after she reached 40. She wrote a book of her experiences that was made into a serial, "Out on a Limb" (1987), for national television. She sought friends to teach her about expanded states of consciousness, read transpersonal literature, and went to psychics who guided her development. She had no other impetus except her own deep desire to learn more. Her support community consisted of one friend who helped her maintain a positive attitude, showed her a map of the journey, and helped her explore new ways of being.

MacLaine's story (1984, 1987) is one well-publicized model of a path which has been independent of the more traditional ways of inviting new ways of being. In the past, people seeking transpersonal levels of development would surrender themselves to monastic life, divesting themselves of their former identities. In monastic life they would do spiritual exercises designed to guide them toward spiritual experiences and transpersonal development. This system was hierarchical. A teacher or abbot had authority over the monastic's life.

Other ways of inviting new ways of being include large group events such as EST and Lifespring, group marathons which are designed to enable people to realize deeper parts of their nature. EST, in particular, has innovated many types of programs to help people push limitations around self-concept and develop new ways to be in the world. Jean Houston's groups are designed to help people see "New Possibilities" for being.

Therapy which is transpersonally oriented is designed to help people develop and experience new possibilities for themselves in all aspects of their lives. It is oriented towards increased well-being. It invites clients to adventure, to explore new ways of being in the world which would increase satisfaction.

Community Resources

The community resources available to you as a Helper are an important part of your professional care of clients in spiritual emergency. In Appendix 'A' of this manual are a questionnaire and discussion guide of community resources. Reading and responding to this will help you and your group identify community resources for referral.

Summary

Supporting people in spiritual emergency is a humanistic art based on compassion and kindness mixed with the technologies of clinical psychology and theology. As we become more aware of the needs of people entering into this critical phase, we will be better prepared to care for them. At this point, we have identified basic elements most necessary to address: a safe environment, grounding, restructuring inhibiting response patterns, and supporting spiritual emergence. Next is a discussion on the role of the Helper.

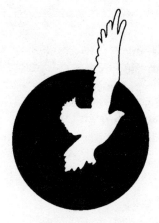

Chapter Six _____

The Role of The Helper

This chapter is designed to assist you to identify your competencies as a Helper. A list of competencies is given, followed by a description of the qualities listed. At the end of the chapter questions are asked to help you review.

Because the list of competencies in an ideal Helper is long, it would be highly unusual to find all qualifications in one person. As you read the following list, keep in mind that the ideal helper may be a team of people, not just one person.

Competencies of a Helper

1. An open heart, compassion.
2. Experience of opening to the Divine.
3. A modicum of clinical experience with people having symptoms of psychosis.
4. Substantial experience with one's own unconscious, including the psychic and astral levels.
5. Groundedness.
6. Stability within oneself.
7. Knowledge and skill in working with body-mind aspects of spiritual emergency.
8. Committment to excellence in one's work.
9. Access to excellent supervision.
10. Knowledge of literature on spiritual emergence.
11. Ability to teach someone about spiritual emergence.
12. Knowledge of one's own skills and when to make referrals.
13. Knowledge of caring for one's own needs.

An Open Heart

An open heart, the ability to be present with compassion, is the most important qualification for a Helper of someone in spiritual emergency. More than anything else, it is the open heartedness of the Helper that is essential for any kind of healing or balancing to happen for the client.

The Experience of Opening to the Divine

A person who has already had a spiritual experience can give reassurance to a person in spiritual crisis. People who have had an opening to the Divine embody a knowingness of the Divine. This deep personal knowledge and the ability to reassure clients about spiritual experience are important characteristics of a Helper.

Clinical Experience

Clinical experience with psychotic clients is essential for the Helper who carries the responsibility of making a correct diagnosis. This experience gives a Helper the skills to work with someone in a psychotic state.

A person with this clinical experience can determine how much and what kind of assistance a client needs, if and when it's safe to leave a client alone, and if the client is sufficiently grounded to get along without assistance.

Experience With One's Own Unconscious

Having a familiarity with the unconscious implies that a Helper has "confronted his [or her] own demons and become conscious of the psychic and astral levels within himself [or herself]" (S. Grof, Oct. 1985). With this familiarity comes a respect for the unconscious and, relatively speaking, less fear in dealing with it. A Helper who has

135

worked with the unconscious is able to provide a client in spiritual emergency with a workable strategy, a model, for relating to unconscious material as it arises.

A Helper who has a deep familiarity with his or her own unconcious is less likely to become destabilized by the eruptions that may come from the unconscious of a client. In helping someone in spiritual emergency, an ability to work with the dark, or shadow side of transpersonal experiences is just as important as the ability to accept and work with the transpersonal or higher aspects of the unconscious.

> *My experience as a trainer of counselors is that a lot of people have had religious awakenings but sometimes they haven't been connected with any aspect of the shadow side of life. The tendency with a therapist is to only give what one understands, and with therapies of the heart, the therapist is the frame that we have. If a person starts to confront their dark side, especially in some dramatic way, where there is movement happening and some sort of abreaction occurring, counselors tend to stop that process, unless they've been willing to go through it themselves. Sometimes they don't stop it consciously, because they know they've been trained not to, yet you will pick up a vibration from them, like "Well, that's enough, now." You'll notice they'll start manipulating the body, sometimes doing bodywork techniques or moving in with an intervention that may accomplish a therapeutic goal for the person at the time, but it has stopped their process.*
>
> (*Small, Oct.1985*)

Another benefit of a Helper who is intimately familiar with the unconscious is that the Helper may have greater familiarity with dreams, archetypal themes, and symbols. This knowledge may be of help to a client in interpreting a dream, creating a meaningful ritual, or sharing a vision. A Helper who is fully aware of his or her own (and others') unconscious material can contribute in a number of meaningful ways to a client developing a strategy for dealing with the unconscious.

Groundedness

A Helper needs to recognize whether he or she is grounded and, if not, how to become grounded. Without such knowledge, the Helper cannot be a stabilizing influence in a spiritual emergency, nor a dependable member of a team of Helpers.

It is not necessary to be grounded all the time. To become close to someone in spiritual emergency, a Helper may need to become relatively ungrounded for a time to match the client. This can be reassuring for the client. However, the Helper in this situation must be able to recognize when he or she is ungrounded and be able to become grounded at will. The client also needs to learn how to move from grounded to ungroundedness and back. The Helper is a model and teacher for this.

Stability Within Oneself

Being stable within oneself means having a stable self-structure, a stable identity. A stable person can withstand being challenged physically, emotionally, and intellectually and not "go to pieces." This does not imply that he or she is "together" all the time, invulnerable or emotionally detached.

One of the most important aspects of being stable is recognizing when you are unstable. Each us is in the process of growing all the time. Although Helpers need to have achieved a level of mature ego development (using Wilber's model in Chapter One), there will be times when the Helper is relatively unstable as part of normal growth. It is essential that the Helper recognize these periods and receive stabilizing support.

A stabilizing force in my life are the weekly staff meetings at the Counseling Center where I work. In addition to helping with client-related problems, these meetings serve to provide support for each of us in our personal lives. We teach each other about the difficulty of being therapists—of having to maintain a supporter role for clients when we, as therapists, may be feeling at sea. We teach each other ways to tolerate these periods and provide support to one another in hard times. It eases the weight of the role of Helper to acknowledge that we are together in this process of growth.

Knowledge and Skill in Bodywork

A skilled bodyworker is an important member on a team of people helping those in spiritual emergency. The type of bodywork is not important—whether for grounding, catalyzing emotional catharsis, or balancing subtle energies. Most important is the ability of such a Helper to articulate the somatic aspects of psychological disturbance.

Recognizing somatic manifestations of spiritual emergency is helpful for diagnosis as well as planning for treatment. For example, many of my clients have transpersonal experiences but have trouble staying grounded. These people lose their sense of priorities; they have trouble steadily working toward a goal; they have difficulty standing up for themselves when challenged. The somatic manifestations of these psychological problems are weak ankles, tight shoulders and neck, and a retracted pelvis. When I see this pattern in the body, I already know that person under stress loses a sense of boundaries and self definition and becomes uncertain or hypersensitive in relationship to others. I know he or she likes spiritual experiences and needs grounding. I also know that as the person gains flexibility in the neck and pelvic areas and strength in the ankles through process oriented body work he or she will become more grounded and more able to integrate on-going spiritual experiences. This kind of information is useful to both clients and other Helpers who are not as familiar with somatic therapies.

Commitment to Excellence

If I were in spiritual emergency, I would want to be with a Helper who was committed to doing an excellent job. When I choose a team to work with, I choose people who are committed to excellence. I learn from them. I can depend on them. I am inspired by them. Isn't that so for all of us?

Access to Excellent Supervision

A good supervisor is an inspiring model as a Helper and can be a lifesaver. A good supervisor helps us in our own growth as well as watching to see if we are appropriately caring for our clients.

Novice Helpers might overlook some very important aspect of their client's lives—especially in times of spiritual crisis. For instance, a novice Helper might be far more involved with some fantastic transpersonal experience than a suicidal idea that may be presented by a client. The Helper might find it easier to talk to the client about God than to ask him if he has any thoughts of suicide. The supervisor's role is to see that the Helper is working with the suicidal ideation as well as the uplifting images of God, modifying treatment to address both the symptoms of depression as well as spiritual emergency.

Knowledge of the Literature of Spiritual Emergence

The Helper who has a good intellectual understanding of spiritual emergence is a valuable advisor to a Helper who does a diagnosis because he or she is less prone to confuse the phenomena of spiritual emergency with psychopathology. Also, this Helper can be a reassuring advisor to clients in spiritual emergency who are looking for an understanding of what is happening to them.

Ability to Teach About Spiritual Emergence

The transpersonal level of experience is difficult to talk about because it involves phenomena that can not be adequately described in words. In addition, many people are highly skeptical about spiritual experiences and are not receptive to learning about something which might challenge their ideas.

A client who holds a traditional scientific perspective of reality may be petrified with fear that he or she is crazy. The Helper must be able to teach the client a positive conceptual framework for his or her experiences.

Sometimes the family of a client in spiritual emergency is determined not to accept the authenticity of spiritual experiences. The ability to teach this family to respect the value of spiritual emergence may be the ingredient that convinces them not to hospitalize their son for schizophrenia, but to explore an alterative diagnostic and treatment procedure. In this example, the Helper

141

who can teach about spiritual emergence has a big responsibility.

The Helper who can teach about spiritual emergence is also important in interfacing with doctors, priests, and other support members in the community who may have an impact on a client's life.

Knowledge of One's Own Skills and When to Make Referrals

> *"It's important to know what you know and it's even more important to know what you don't know."*
>
> *(Roberts,1973)*

A Helper needs to know his or her skills and limitations so that referrals to others can be made, as necessary, for the comprehensive care of the client. For example, a Helper trained in verbal therapy may want to bring a bodyworker in to assist with a client. A Helper who is a bodyworker may need to cooperate with a medical doctor about a client's care, and so on.

Knowing How to Care for One's Own Needs

Perhaps the most important skill of the Helper is providing for his or her own well-being. Helpers, as well as clients, need on-going support for their personal growth and well-being.

Helpers need to identify their own needs for rest and retreat, for play, physical exercise, and proper nourishment, close contact with friends and family, and activities in which other interests are pursued. Helpers need to also have cultivated their own connections with a community, a network of friends, a religious institution or teacher that support their spiritual unfolding. Helpers serve as models of well-being to their clients in spiritual emergency. The Helper's ability to provide for his own well-being thus serves not only himself but his clients.

Assess Your Competencies

Following is a list of questions you can use to assess your competencies in helping people in spiritual emergency. You may find it helpful to reflect on these by yourself, and subsequently in discussion with your peer group.

1. Do I want to be a Helper? Do I feel compassion for and interest in people in spiritual emergency?

2. What kind of experiences have I had in the Subtle and Causal levels? What kind of support am I capable of giving to another person opening up in this area?

3. What clinical experience have I had? Have I worked with people who are clinically psychotic? Have I been with people who were in spiritual emergency?

4. What are my skills in doing experiential bodywork with people? How much experience have I had? At what point would I refer a client to someone else in transpersonal bodywork or breathwork?

5. How comfortable do I feel with my own shadow, with the dark elements of myself? Have I met my grief, my rage, my fear, my sexuality, my ecstasy, my power? Have I been around paranormal events? Have I seen visions? Have I experienced kundalini? Have I experienced other forms of spiritual emergency?

6. Do I feel grounded at this time in my life? Do I know how to get grounded when I feel out of balance? What do I do to get grounded? What can I teach other people to do? Can I perform well in highly stressful situations? Do I know when to say "No" and how to care for my own personal needs?

7. Do I feel a strong sense of connection with energies larger than my own ego that are positive and universal?

8. Do I have support/ supervision which will back me up in my work as a Helper? Who are these people?

9. What is my knowledge of psychological literature to help me differentiate between psychological disturbance and spiritual emergency? What is my knowledge of spiritual texts? Can this knowledge be applied to other's spiritual experiences?

10. Whom am I most suited to help?

11. What do I know of other people who are working in this area as Helpers? What do I know of their work? Do I feel comfortable referring client's to them? What self-help groups and spiritually oriented communities do I know? What do I know of their work? Can I refer people to them? Do I feel comfortable with referring people to them? Who makes referrals to me?

References for Helpers

Following is a list of books which I have found to be helpful in exploring the role of a Helper:

Da Free John, <u>The Dawn Horse Testament</u>. San Rafael, CA.: Dawn Horse Press, 1985.

Guggenbuhl-Craig, A., <u>Power and the Helping Professions</u>, Irving, Texas: Spring, 1971.

Grof, S., <u>Beyond the Brain,</u> Albany, New York: State University of New York, 1985.

Hendricks, G. and Weinhold, B.,<u>Transpersonal Approaches to Counseling and Psychotherapy,</u> Denver, Colorado: Love, 1982.

Kopp,S., <u>Back to One</u>, Palo Alto, California: Science and Behavior Books, 1977.

Perry,J.W.,<u>The Far Side of Madness,</u> New Jersey: Prentice Hall, 1974.

Ram Dass and Gorman, P., <u>How Can I Help?,</u> New York: Knopf, 1985.

Small, J., <u>Transformers:The Therapists of the Future,</u> California: De Vorss & Co., 1982.

Speeth, K.R., *On Psychotherapeutic Attention*. The Journal of Transpersonal Psychology, 1982, 14(2), pp. 141-160.

Wilber, K., No Boundary, Boulder, Colorado: Shambhala, 1981.

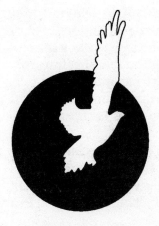

Chapter Seven ────────────────────────────

A Case Study

The following case study is the story of my mother, age 56, and myself at age 24 as we went through a period of intense spiritual experiences in 1971.

My mother, Marjorie, was living alone in a small Vermont town, working as a visiting nurse and practicing Zen Buddhist meditation 6-8 hours a day. She had no affiliation with a church at that time, although previously she had been Unitarian. She had separated from my father in 1964, 7 years prior, and he lived several hundreds of miles away as did all of her three children including me.

My mother had experienced periods of depression during her life and had occasional heart palpitations that at times inhibited her activities. She resisted any form of medication or psychotherapy although she inwardly feared she might have inherited her mother's manic-depressive disorder. Marjorie paid attention to her diet and exercise and was basically in good health.

I was not aware of any particular psycho-social stressors other than the normal anxieties of middle age. Although we were not particularly close, she was planning to visit me to help with the birth of my first child, expected in a couple of months.

Her immediate personal support came from the local general practitioner and a few companions who lived close by, none of whom were involved in Zen Buddhism. The two people she regarded as spiritual teachers lived hundreds of miles from her home.

Her closest friend was alarmed because Marjorie sequestered herself for such long periods of time in meditation, and seemed to be more emotional than was typical for her. This woman had called my brother about her concern, and was trying to do what she could to bring Marjorie to a more normal frame of mind.

One day Marjorie went up into the woods alone. She was reading a passage from <u>Zen Mind, Beginner's Mind</u> (Suzuki, 1970), which related enlightenment to physical death. When she was found dead, she still had her finger marking the page. She had cut her wrist and throat, and died.

Her suicide was a great shock to our family and friends. It was totally unexpected. We had all assumed she was getting along quite well, despite some depression and spending a great deal of time alone. She had been taking trips and she was very active with her work as a visiting nurse.

My husband walked into the house in the middle of the day and told me he had heard some bad news. I was in the midst of doing relaxation exercises in preparation for childbirth. When he told me my mother was dead the shock catapulted me into an intense period of spiritual and psychological experiences which were confusing, overwhelming and enlightening simultaneously.

Fortunately, the Zen Center community, of which I had been a member for several years and Suzuki Roshi himself served as Helpers for me. Suzuki was deeply compassionate, present, and non-judgmental. He was also willing to extend himself on my behalf. He flew with my husband and me to Vermont to lead the traditional Buddhist funeral ceremony at my mother's home. My brother and sister felt this was appropriate. Two of my dearest friends in the Zen community joined us. Their support helped me come to terms with the profound issues surrounding my mother's suicide.

The love and compassion I experienced buffered me from the abysmal loneliness and fear typically felt by people in spiritual emergency. The philosophical understanding I received from Buddhist writings, my spiritual teacher, Suzuki Roshi, and ritual gave me a structure to help comprehend my mother's death, and my own transpersonal experiences.

The transpersonal experiences began when my husband, who knew none of the details of her death, told me my mother had died. I sobbed in grief for a few minutes. Then, a tremendous peace came over me. Starting at my toes, I felt liquid light fill my body, up through the top of my head accompanied by a sense of ecstatic release. I felt sure, at the time, that I was experiencing what my mother had gone through. In a flash, I realized that she was fine and that her passing had been a happy occasion for her. I realized those of us who were left would go through a period of darkness, of doubt, missing her, and wondering if we were at fault in any way. But, I knew in that moment, in every cell of my body, that there was no blame to anyone, and that she was happy. Then, my consciousness returned to grieving and feeling her loss, but I retained the inner knowingness of her happiness. I felt I had in some way experienced her death with her.

The experience of feeling her presence did not continue with the same intensity, however I still felt unusually close to what was happening with her. I felt a quality of bliss and release I had never experienced before in my life. I sensed she had become one with all things, and , at the same time, although bodily gone, was still present as herself.

My subjective experience of her death was confirmed by her friend who found her who told me that mother had a smile lighting her face when she died.

After the funeral, when my family and friends sat with Suzuki Roshi in conversation, someone asked, "Where did Marjorie go when she died?" He said, " She did not go anywhere. She is a part of the grass, the trees, the sky, the brook. She is here with us and, she is everywhere."

After the funeral I became preoccupied with my own questions. How did I know that she was happy? How did I retain the sense of where she was? How could I know these things so certainly? Was I deluding myself out of the stress of the experience? My inner preoccupation continued for weeks. I wondered if I was a bit crazy. Finally, when I had gone 10 days past my delivery date, I began to worry that something was wrong. I went to my garden to pray and made an internal commitment to stop questioning myself about my mother for now and until two months after the birth. Within an hour, the contractions started and eight hours later my son was born. Two months later, I saw a spiritual teacher who validated my experience of knowing what was happening with my mother. She told me that I was having a series of Subtle and Causal level experiences (although she didn't use those terms). She confirmed that I wasn't crazy. She encouraged me to continue to be receptive to these experiences.

There were many sources of support during that period when I thought I was going crazy...rituals, friends, family, and the beauty of the Vermont countryside. Suzuki Roshi performed a succession of rituals around the death which lasted several days and included prayers to guide my mother's soul into her next life. My friends and family shared these rituals. One included a procession to the funeral at the top of the hill, to a place we had gathered for picnics. I sounded a bell every few steps. My husband carried the ashes in a ceramic pot I had made.

It was a very touching ceremony that we created. At one point during the funeral, I dissolved in tears. Sadness, anger, confusion, and doubts had overwhelmed me. I wondered what was real, I felt confused about my becoming a mother when my mother had just died. Even though I had the deep knowingness in the background that she had transmitted her bliss to me, I wondered, like a child, where she was. I let myself feel all the instinctual feelings that are part of deep grief. My friends and family did not intrude, or withdraw. They allowed me my grieving, bless their souls.

The beauty of the Vermont countryside also helped me. It seemed to absorb my pain and reaffirm my faith that life would be abundant and peace would return.

All these resources—my Zen community, Suzuki Roshi, the rituals, my friends and family, and Vermont's natural beauty, prevented my period of grief from becoming an unbearable crisis. Additionally, I had developed an ability to deal with deep emotional and spiritual experiences through my own spiritual practice and Reichian therapy.

My experience might not have been so positive had I not understood intellectually what was going on, had no philosophical background to guide my understanding, had no person who was compassionate or understood what was happening to me, felt alone or felt afraid of the overpowering spiritual, emotional, and physical experiences, or felt unsupported in expressing myself emotionally or creatively.

My mother had not benefitted from support as I had. My belief is that she took her life in a misunderstanding that physical death would bring her the enlightenment experience for which she yearned. If a spiritual teacher or a competent Helper had been close by, she most likely would not have fallen into this delusion . She may have been, instead, guided into some inner work that would have been life-affirming, empowering her spiritual emergence in life.

Although both my mother and I had spiritual experiences that resulted in spiritual emergency, only I received the excellent support required to integrate the experience in a life-affirming way. This story is a dramatic illustration of the value of Helpers.

Nirvana, the Waterfall-

Our life and death are the same thing. When we realize this fact, we have no fear of death anymore, nor actual difficulty in our life....When the water returns to its original oneness with the river, it no longer has any individual feeling to it; it resumes its own nature, and finds composure. How very glad the water must be to come back to the original river !

....That is why we say, "To attain Nirvana is to pass away." "To pass away" is not a very adequate expression. Perhaps "to pass on," or "to go on," or "to join" would be better. Will you try to find some better expression for death?

(Suzuki, 1970)

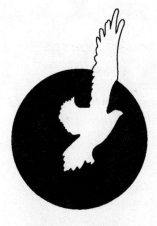

Chapter Eight ———————————————

Global Trends
Catalyzing Spiritual Emergence

This chapter describes major social and scientific changes
that are impelling people all over the world to reflect
deeply on the nature of their lives and to actively
participate in the evolution of life on earth. In essence, we
are being forced to grow to higher levels of consciousness,
to become more mature in order to handle the
responsibilities demanded by the times. Increased tempo
of change and increased self-awareness are two catalysts
for spiritual emergence on a global scale.

Increased Tempo of Change

*Never before has a product of evolution partic-
ipated so actively in accelerating the evolutionary
process. Here are just a few examples...within the
last decades biologists have learned how to modify
the genes in a cell, opening the door to the creation
of completely new species. Now new life-forms
can be designed consciously and created
rapidly...with the advent of particle accelerators,
scientists...are now able to change some elements
into others, or even create completely new elements,
by bombarding the nucleus with atomic particles
and thereby changing its structure...we have
created a fundamentally new way of directly
harnessing the sun's energy: the solar cell. This
invention represents an evolutionary development
as significant as that of photosynthesis 3.5 billion
years ago.*

(Russell, 1983, p.72-4)

*Jumps by so many orders of magnitude, in so many
areas, with the unprecedented coincidence of several
jumps at the same time, and these unique
disturbances of the planet, surely indicate that we
are not passing through a smooth cyclical or
acceleration process similar to those in the historical
past. Anyone who is willing to admit that there
have been sudden jumps in evolution or human
history, such as the invention of agriculture or the
Industrial Revolution, must conclude from this*

evidence that we are passing through another such jump far more concentrated and more intense than these, and of far greater evolutionary importance.

(John Platt, "The Futurist" as cited in Russell, 1983)

Two of the most important innovations in science and technology are improved communications and increased mobility, both of which have accelerated the growth of knowledge around the world. In this century we have moved from cars travelling 15 miles per hour to supersonic rockets travelling at 25,000 miles per hour. We have progressed from radio broadcasting to television satellite linkups—increasing significantly the quantity, quality, and availability of information.

Sharing knowledge among nations has greatly increased, with dramatic consequences. This has led to better health care, increased production, higher standards of living, and more efficient land use-factors that have enabled the population to grow faster. In fact, the human population is now growing at a superexponential rate; in the 1960's, it was doubling every 35 years (Russell, 1983). Increasingly more people share a high standard of living with time to reflect on themselves and to network with people all over the world.

International communications have allowed for a cross-fertilization of ideas, attitudes, and values affecting the quality of our inner lives just as international monetary trade and technology exchange have affected the quality of our outer lives. Many of us have learned that the

Russian people are as interested in international peace as the American people. Many of us have learned about the variety of religious practices, medical practices, and cultural patterns in the world. Many of us have come to realize that we have far more in common with others than we have differences.

Above all, the longing for peace and well-being in the world in the face of terrorism and nuclear meltdowns has created a deep bond amongst many people, felt all the more strongly as more people discover that human beings now have the power to destroy all life on this planet in a matter of minutes by the explosion of nuclear warheads.

Not only is there accelerated growth in communication, travel, and population but some of our most stable social institutions are breaking down. As Harman (1985) pointed out, Americans have put more and more energy into stabilizing our economic and defense systems, and have, ironically, produced unwieldy deficits, and incalculable risks to our security because of nuclear warheads which must be managed faultlessly or else lead to global destruction. The institutions of finance and defense in the United States are no longer a witness, guard, or even symbol of our stability as a nation. The social order of Caucasian male domination has been dismantled by the civil rights and women's movements. This is a state, as Tofler put it, of "future shock".

One of the most dynamic changes in our perception of reality has been suggested by physicists - especially those who study particle physics. Just as Ptolemy initiated the Copernican revolution by suggesting that the earth rotated around the sun, so today some physicists have initiated a crisis by proving that the observer has a dynamic relationship to the observed - the observer modifies the thing observed by his or her expectations and attitudes. Thus, it is now possible to say with some proof that what we study is inseparable from who we are. Some physicists have thus demonstrated in physical terms the content of a Causal experience - the inseparableness of all things, the unity of all things, that life is determined by consciousness itself, which cannot be seen, observed ojectively, or quantified. These thoughts go beyond all usual collective attitudes about the nature of the world.

This new understanding of the nature of reality, the acceleration of information and technological change, and the simultaneous breakdown of our most powerful social institutions is bringing on a crisis of momentous proportions-especially in the population of high technology cultures (Harman,1985). And, because our world has grown into a hierarchical structure with the rich and powerful commanding the most resources and making decisions which determine the quality of life of the not-so-rich, the most well educated people are the first to experience this crisis. What we do will have a major impact on the rest of the world. So, what do we do?

Those people who hang on to the old perspective - that reality is only that which can be seen and measured - and those people who hang onto the old social institutions for stability may find it increasingly difficult to understand their world. Those people who choose to become conscious of and accepting of a new reality are the ones emerging into a "global consciousness" (Harman, 1985). Global consciousness is integral to spiritual emergence in that it is premised on the unitary nature of all things. People caught in the middle of the new and the old realities may find themselves in spiritual emergency, incapable of integrating the new perspective. Their old realities are shattering and they are attempting to make way for the new reality which demands more self awareness and a deepening sense of one's true nature.

Television, radio and newspapers constantly bombard us with pictures and stories of events and people around the world—in a way forcing a global consciousness on anyone who listens. In the mid 1980's people who are aware of the news have become aware of the starvation of whole nations in Africa, the earthquakes of Mexico, the carnage of political civil wars in South America, and so on. This awareness of the chaotic state of our world creates a catalyst toward spiritual emergence as educated and sensitive people feel the need to respond on an ever-more highly conscious level to the world situation (Cappadonna, 1985; Lindberg, 1955).

> *We are the world,*
> *We are the children*
> *We are the ones who make a brighter day*
> *So let's start giving*
> *There's a choice we're making*
> *We're saving our own lives*
> *It's true we'll make a better day*
> *Just you and me.*

> *(United Support of Artists for Africa, 1985)*

A new level of awareness of world views other than the Western Christian-Judeo perspective has also resulted from greater communication and mobility.

Cross-fertilization of Religious Practices

> *In the west we have generally accepted the concretization of the world. We see it as really something solid and permanent. This has been built on since the development of sciences and Cartesianism. The contradiction of the inner realization of the dreamlike quality of reality to the outer world's belief system is an enormous conflict to live with. Without a supportive philosophy and supportive friends, persons undergoing the awakening in the West might well assume they are going crazy as they have nothing to support their experience as real and positive. This realization is not as difficult for a traditional Buddhist to accept because he has recognized this as truth from the time he first heard the Buddhist teachings.*
>
> *(Sogyal, 1985)*

As Buddhist and other Eastern practices become more available in the West, some Westerners have found them supportive in transforming their experience of reality to include "global consciousness" and transpersonal states of consciousness.

Sogyal Rinpoche is one of the Eastern religious leaders who has helped introduce Eastern religious ideas in the West. Sogyal is an incarnate Lama, a scholar, and a meditation master. He was born in Tibet, the son of one of the greatest Buddhist masters of this century. Sogyal left Tibet when it was invaded by China in the 1950's. He studied at Cambridge University and has now lived and taught Buddhism for more than 12 years in the West. The Tibetans' evacuation from their country and subsequent absorption into other areas of the world has made Tibetan Buddhism accessible to many cultures.

Other non-western religions have also moved into the stream of Western culture in the last century as a result of political shifts and increased mobility between cultures. Many Eastern mystics and religious leaders had been introduced in the West before the latter half of the 1900s (for example,Yogananda, Alice Bailey, Krishnamurti, and Graf von Durkheim). It wasn't until the baby-boomers born after World War II became teens in the 1960's, however, that Eastern religions and religious practices (Transcendental Meditation and Zen especially) were popularized. Today, evidence that the realities proposed by Eastern religions are becoming integrated with Western perspectives can be seen in Western literature (Zen and the Art of Motorcycle Maintenance, Pirsig,1979), movies (The Karate Kid, I and II), spiritual teachers like Brother David Steindl-Rast who incorporates Eastern meditation techniques into devotional Catholic monastic life, and the popularity of the practice of martial arts, Hatha Yoga, and T'ai Chi for relaxation and exercise.

Cross-fertilization of Medical Practices

Like religious practices, Eastern medical technologies which substantiate the new reality have also had a widespread effect on Western culture.

Eastern medical approaches, such as Chinese acupuncture and Tibetan Ayurvedic medicine, see the body as a dance of elemental energies which are constantly in flux, constantly influencing the energetic balance of each organ system. Eastern medical perspectives diagnose imbalances in the body by taking into account both concrete, physical events as well as non-physical processes.

> *Tibetan medicine looks very much into what is called prana, the wind, the inner wind...when the wind goes through different channels it creates different experiences. When the wind goes into the heart area then it begins to create some kind of very (spiritually powerful opening) experiences...even some of the Lamas have grave wind element.*

> *(Sogyal, May 1985)*

"Prana" is like a spiritual force which comes from what Westerners might call heaven. It is an energy which, combined with the heart, can uplift and purify the emotional nature of any person. Thus, it is a force which can create profound experience.

In diagnosing and treating people who are involved in spiritual emergency it is particularly important to look at the way Subtle energies are moving in their bodies (Raheem, 1985). Movement toward greater awareness in the mind creates a shift in the energies of the body. Balancing of energy must be done by someone who understands both the physical body processes as well as Subtle energies. These techniques are not taught in the medical schools of the West but come through the traditions associated with Chinese medicine, including Chinese herbal medicine, Ayurvedic medicine, and some of the practices coming from the ancient Yogic traditions of India.

These ancient systems of looking at the body, diagnosing illness and treating imbalance have an inherent belief that human beings are expressions of the elemental forces which are part of all nature. These systems teach the value of attuning to subtle energies in the body so as to feel more palpably akin to life and more able to sense our connection with the highest energy, the Divine.

Heidegger, the German philosopher, stated this concept of what it is to be a human being in the following way: "A person is neither a thing nor a process, but an opening or a clearing through which the Absolute can manifest" (personal communication to K. Wilber, cited in Vaughan, 1986).

This point of view, prevalent in the medical practices of the East, has had a profound effect on many Western health practitioners. The number of people turning to the Wholistic Health movement in the West is also a sign of the success and acceptance of the Eastern approaches to health maintenance.

Increased Self Awareness Through the Use of Drugs

Drug use has been a dual-edged sword for our society— at the same time as it has been the catalyst for destruction for some, for others it has opened a world of new perspective and increased meaning.

Drug use has been epidemic in the West in the last two decades. This is a by-product of our increased international trade, mobility and more sophisticated technology. Drugs come to us from all over the world, including our own well-equipped laboratories.

The fact that the irresponsible use of drugs has thrown users into lives of ill health and self destruction is well known; less recognized are the potentially positive aspects of the so-called "recreational drugs" which can catalyze self healing and spiritual experience. Some drugs, when used in a therapeutic setting, are shown to increase sensitivity, creativity, empathy and compassion. Thus, these drugs may potentiate spiritual emergence, and they may indicate one way to increase self awareness.

A few researchers are investigating the responsible use of "recreational" drugs for their therapeutic effects.

Strassman (1984) reviewed the literature on the potentially beneficial psychological effects of psychedelics used in a therapeutic setting and suggests that it is time to begin to investigate how they might be used legally.

> *...a decade of inactivity in this area of research has given us the necessary time to reflect on what has been learned and what needs further investigation. The relative roles of set and setting, motivations for drug use, personal and family history of mental illness, defensive style, and level of object relatedness, should all be used in careful selection, screening, and preparation of subjects for psychedelic research. It appears that, if these factors are carefully controlled, the incidence of acute and more long term problems associated with their use can be kept to a minimum. The benefits that can be obtained in terms of an increased knowledge of psychedelic drug-induced altered mental states, and their potential therapeutic roles, seems to justify these risks.*
>
> *(Strassman, 1984, p.592)*

MDMA, (Ecstasy), when used in a therapeutic setting, has also proven to have significant value in opening people to psychological healing and spiritual emergence.

> *Four psychiatrists who use MDMA in clinical practice reported on the findings of more than 1,000 sessions at a recent California conference sponsored by the Earth Metabolic Design Laboratory.*

Their overall conclusions, as phrased in an article in press. "The reports of MDMA's facilitation of psychotherapy were impressive. Many subjects experienced classic retrieval of lost traumatic memories, followed by relief of emotional symptoms."

...Psychiatrist George Greer concluded that his study of 29 patients demonstrated "a potential use for MDMA as a safe and effective adjunct to therapy especially for the prevention and treatment of interpersonal problems and substance use disorders."

The most common benefits: improved communication and intimacy between family members and couples. Aftereffects included higher self-esteem, positive mood and a decreased use of addictive substances.

Most subjects reported an expanded mental perspective or insight. Several said they felt undesirable emotional symptoms such as anxiety during the sessions and sadness afterward. Five described transcendent experiences.

All nine with specific psychiatric disorders reported significant relief from their problems. Two said they had full and lasting remissions.

(Brain Mind Bulletin, April,1985)

Further research may substantiate that psychedelics and empathogens, **when used in a therapeutic or religious setting,** are powerful tools to help people open to and feel more secure in the realities of a more expanded consciousness.

Ideally, we could then decide to return to a time when:

> *abuse (of drugs) apparently was fairly rare, perhaps because careful cultural, religious, and social proscriptions determined a uniform manner in which these substances were used and the experiences one was expected to have as a result of their use.*
>
> *(A. Weil, 1972)*

The opportunity to explore the potential benefits of these drugs that have often been misused by an uneducated and unprepared public will be affected by research monies and political opinion.

Summary

Alternative medical systems are challenging the authority of our traditional medical institutions, the new physics is challenging the authority of traditional scientific views. Global consciousness is challenging nationalism. Altered states of consciousness brought on through drugs and/ or meditation practices are giving those who experience them new perceptions of who they are. Headlines declare that the institution of the family is crumbling and that Christian churches are losing favor with many young people. The political authority of the world leaders is challenged by violent assassinations and political scandal. This is the evidence visible to people aware of the world situation that we are involved in The Dark Night of the Ego, a deep identity crisis brought on by our varied attempts to cope with tumultuous change.

This time of upheaval has intensified self-inquiry by many individuals and nations. It has made many people push against the limits of their own developmental level. Under the stress of meeting a constantly accelerating change in reality, some of these people (and countries) will break into pieces in their own kind of spiritual emergency, others will move more flexibly in their developmental processes.

Individuals and nations grow; and there is a collective global growth process, too. All people on this globe may be in the process of expanding to a level of self-structure beyond the ordinary bounds of ego, or national identity. This level may have more to do with self-actualized spirit than the ordinary kinds of self-centered organizations that have heretofore made up our identity structures. The end point could possibly parallel a transpersonal level of consciousness for an individual on a larger scale—a global community which has found a way to live in harmony, sharing material well-being, radiating peace, creativity and joy.

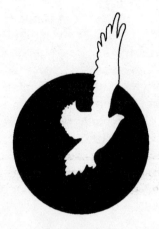

Chapter Nine —————————————————

Suggestions for the Future of the Spiritual Emergence Network

At the SEN invited conferences in May and and October,1985 several discussions focused on future plans for SEN. The suggestions from the participants covered the areas of education, research, referral and a 24 hour care center.

Education

In the future we would like to host large conferences in the San Francisco Bay Area on themes associated with spiritual emergence. This would give people who have been interested in the small Esalen conferences a chance to meet other professionals in the field, to exchange ideas, and to be inspired by others' work.

One suggestion was to dialogue by computer with people in other parts of the world as part of a conference. This would enable them to be in close touch with our discussions in the Bay Area and to give us immediate and interactive feedback. Such computerized meta-networking would speed communications dramatically and strengthen the connections between our SEN centers world-wide.

Interest was shown in the development of workshops training Helpers. The workshops could be presented to specific communities worldwide to enable them to learn about spiritual emergence and working with people in spiritual emergency.

A suggestion was made to develop a library, open to SEN members, for materials related to spiritual emergence and helping people in spiritual emergency.

Research

Many studies were suggested as potentially valuable such as; 1) The effect of drug vs. non-drug treatment for people in spiritual emergency, 2) The effect of environment in the treatment of people in spiritual emergency, and 3) Defining appropriate tools for diagnosis.

There are many other areas that need to be researched. There is a particular need to study 24 hour treatment centers for spiritual emergency - to determine how one could be set up, how to work with insurance and state funding, and what kind of support team one needs to manage such a facility. Statistics need to be gathered to chronicle treatment given at the facility, and the results gained by clients.

SEN has received support from the Threshhold Foundation and private individuals for the maintenance of networking and educational services. Research into alternative funding sources must be made.

Referral Network

There are now 10,000 people on our mailing list including those who have been inspired by the Grofs, those who have called when they were in need of help, professionals who want to be on our referral list, and many others.

Much of SEN's staff time is spent answering inquiries about SEN's purpose, reducing time to contact Helpers and supporters and to maintain the quality of our referral network. In the future we want to improve our communication with Helpers so that we have the most complete information on hand about their particular talents and competencies for helping people in spiritual emergence and spiritual emergency.

24 Hour Care Facility

A 24-hour-care facility is needed to which we can refer people in spiritual emergency. It is frustrating to have identified the necessary treatment for a person in spiritual emergency and to realize that there is only one facility of this kind available in California, and one other in New Hampshire (see Appendix D).

A 24-hour-care facility is needed near the Menlo Park area. It should be large enough to house at least 6 to 8 clients at first, with accommodations for more in separate dwellings. Each house would function as a small community where members would eat together and live as a family unit. There should be a psychiatrist on staff in a supervisory role. The daily staff would be trained Helpers who are not necessarily licensed by any current licensing standards. These staff would be trained by SEN, and each would have particular skills in working with spiritual emergency including transpersonal bodywork, breathwork, and spiritual practices. The staff would function as members of the household, along with clients, fostering a homelike, egalitarian atmosphere.

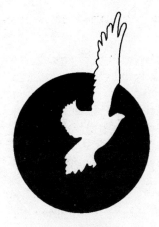

Appendix A

Identifying Community Resources for Helping People in Spiritual Emergency

I suggest first answering the following questions by yourself and then discussing them with other people to get ideas on additional community resources you may not have recognized. You might make notes for your own referral system for future reference.

I.   Joe

You become aware of a man, Joe, who is very upset and is not functioning in his job. He is having visions. He says they are 'visions of God'. He is also afraid he might be going crazy because no one seems to be able to understand him. Joe has no religious context to understand the visions either. He is spending time by himself, and seems to be feeling more and more alientated by people. Joe is also suffering from migraine headaches.

What are your community's resources for helping this person? Consider the following questions:

1. Is there a doctor, psychologist, or paraprofessional who could identify whether Joe is in spiritual emergency and/or whether he needs psychiatric care?

2. Is there a health-care worker who can evaluate the appropriateness of using drugs to help Joe?

3. Is there a retreat where Joe could go to get intensive care and support if he is unable to care for himself? Where is this?

4. Is there a person in the community who can help Joe deal with the energy in the migraine headache, to diagnose its physical cause and/or free the energy blockage? Are there persons in the community skilled in transpersonal

bodywork and /or breathwork? Who are they? Where are they located?

5. Is Joe a member of a religious group? Does this group have the resources to give him guidance? If there is no one in the community of ministers who can help, are there other persons who might be able to give guidance as needed? Who are they? Where are they located? Are they available?

6. What resources are there outside of my community to help in any of the above?

II. Ginny

You become aware of a woman, Ginny, who is reaching out to make friends, wanting to talk about her experience living in an ashram for 4 years. She feels her life has been enriched by the experience, but she now needs to be more in contact with other kinds of people. She is experiencing dreams and paranormal phenomena which lead her to feel as if she has made a mistake in leaving the ashram. Ginny's old friends at the ashram are pressuring her to return, threatening that if she doesn't return she will lose her only chance at becoming enlightened. Ginny often feels depressed, scared and lonely.

What are your community's resources for helping Ginny? Consider her religious background, her current social situation, and her moods. Refer to the numbered questions in case #I for help in reflecting.

III. Jim

A mother calls you to talk about her 13-year-old son, Jim, who has "turned into a different person since being turned on to drugs." When he was younger he used to play alone with his "imaginary friends" but he "got over" that. He became more outgoing and played with other kids. Now, she is worried that Jim won't develop the discipline to get along in life. He's lost interest in school. She doesn't know how to talk to him. She doesn't know anything about what drugs he is taking. Jim is withdrawing more and more from the family. He likes to sit quietly by himself and paint.

1. Who in the community is most prepared to help Jim and Jim's family? Why?

2. Is this just a drug problem? Are there other issues related to Jim's personal development? Who is in the best position to answer this question?

3. What would be the best way to help Jim in his personal development at this stage in his life?

IV. Lyn

Lyn, a woman of 42, calls you. She has been reading
<u>Dancing in the Light</u> by Shirley MacLaine. She wants to
know community resources for learning about her past
lives. Her marriage is breaking up. Lyn has just had a
hysterectomy and has been hospitalized with a pelvic
infection which caused high fevers for several weeks.
She said she had some "bizarre experiences" while she
was sick. She felt she was "leaving her body." She wants
to understand what is happening to her. She feels lonely
and afraid. She feels she can't talk to her doctor or her
minister about any of this. Her husband calls her "crazy."
Lyn has a passion to find out more about these inexplicable
phenomena. "I just have to understand what's happening
to me!"

1. Who in your community could help Lyn with her
   interest in past lives? What kind of help does she
   need?

2. Who in the community could help her understand
   what happened to her when she was sick?

3. Does this woman need continued support? If so,
   what kind, or kinds.

Your Community's Resources

After reflecting on the above situations, list the answers to the following questions regarding your community resources.

1. Who would be best at diagnosis which differentiates between spiritual emergency and psychopathology? What are their specialties?

2. Who offers retreat settings or therapeutic communities to support people who need intensive care or adequate supervision for their religious practices?

3. Who is most knowledgeable about psychiatric drugs and mind-altering drugs? What are their opinions about psychiatric drugs, recreational drugs, or the therapeutic use of drugs?

4. Is there a bodyworker in our community who can help a person work with Subtle energy blockages? If not, where can I locate one?

5. Who would I trust to help me if I were in a spiritual emergency? Why?

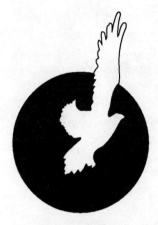

Appendix B ─────────────────────

Evaluating Your Knowledge
of Spiritual Emergency/Emergence

Following is a list of questions to help you reflect on what
you have read in the manual.

   1.   What is spiritual emergence?

   2.   What is spiritual emergency?

   3.   Identify the signs of spiritual emergence.

   4.   Identify the symptoms of psychosis.

5. How do you distinguish between psychosis and spiritual emergence/emergency.

6. Identify six forms of spiritual emergency.

7. Briefly define the Subtle, Causal and Atman levels of human development. Why are they called transpersonal?

8. Do people grow from one developmental level to the next in an orderly progression?

9. Why does progress to transpersonal levels include deeply regressed states ?

10. Identify six personal circumstances that can catalyze spiritual emergence.

11. Identify seven social circumstances that may be catalyzing people towards spiritual emergence on a global scale.

12. Identify five elements of giving on-going support to a person in spiritual emergency.

13. Identify three themes vital to helping someone in spiritual emergence.

14. How many people in the USA have had deep experiences of a transpersonal nature? Why do many people hesitate to talk about their transpersonal experiences?

15. If you were to be a Helper with people in spiritual emergence, how do you imagine yourself working?

After completing these questions, you may want to review parts of the manual for further clarification or to note some of your own reflections on spiritual emergence/emergency.

I would welcome your ideas and thoughts about developing this manual and other educational materials to teach people about spiritual emergence. Please write to me, Emma Bragdon, care of SEN[1] with your suggestions. Thank you.

---

[1] SEN, 250 Oak Grove Ave., Menlo Park, California, 94025

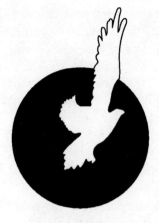

Appendix C ─────────────

Articles of Interest

Forms of Spiritual Emergency
Dr. Stanislav Grof and Christina Grof

All forms of transpersonal crisis can be seen as dynamic exteriorizations of deep unconscious and superconscious realms of the human psyche, which represents one indivisible, multidimensional continuum without any clear boundaries. It is, therefore, obvious that sharp demarcation of various types of spiritual emergency is in practice not possible.

However, we feel on the basis of our work with individuals in spiritual crisis and the study of relevant literature that it is possible and useful to distinguish several major experiential patterns which are particularly frequent. Although they often overlap, each of them has certain characteristic features of its own that differentiate it from others.

I.   Awakening of the Serpent Power (Kundalini)

Although the concept of Kundalini found its most articulate expression in the Indian Tantric tests of Hinduism, Buddhism, Jainism, and in the Tibetan Vajrayana, important parallels can be found in Christian Mysticism, Sufism, Taoist Yoga, Korean Zen, in the freemasonic tradition, among the North American tribes, and the Kung Bushmen of the African Kalihari Desert to name just a few. In a sense, the awakening of Kundalini can be seen as a central mechanism underlying many types of transpersonal crisis.

The ascent of Kundalini as described in the Indian literature can be accompanied by dramatic physical and psychological manifestations called Kriyas. The most striking among these are powerful sensations of heat and energy streaming up the spine, associated with tremors, spasms, violent shaking, and complex twisting movements.

Quite common is involuntary laughing or crying, chanting of mantras or songs, talking in tongues, emitting of vocal noises and animal sounds, and assuming spontaneous yogic gestures (mudras) and postures (asanas). As the Kundalini is freeing physical blockages, the individual can experience intense pain in various parts of the body.

The process of Kundalini awakening can simulate many psychiatric disorders, particularly schizophrenia or other types of psychosis. The presence of characteristic energy phenomena, intense sensations of heat, unusual breathing patterns, pains in characteristic blocking sites for which there is no organic basis, visions of light, and the typical trajectory of the process are among the signs that distinguish the Kundalini syndrome from psychosis.

The individuals involved are also typically much more objective about their condition, communicate and cooperate well, show interest in sharing their experiences with open-minded people, and seldom act out. Although hearing of various sounds is quite common, intruding persecutory voices do not belong to the phenomenology of Kundalini awakening.

II. Shamanic Journey

Transpersonal crises of this type bear a deep resemblance to what the anthropologists have described as the "shamanic" or "initiatory illness." It is a dramatic episode of a non-ordinary state of consciousness that marks the beginning of the career of many shamans. The core experience of the shamanic journey is a profound encounter with death and subsequent rebirth. Initiatory dreams and visions portray a descent into the underworld and exposure to unimaginable tortures.

In the experiences of individuals whose transpersonal crises have strong shamanic features, there is an emphasis on physical suffering and encounter with death followed by rebirth and elements of ascent or magical flight. They typically sense special connection with the elements of nature and experience communication with animals or animal spirits. It is also not unusual to feel an upsurge of special powers and impulses to heal.

Shamanism is practically universal; its varieties can be found in Siberia and other parts of Asia, in North and South America, Australia, Oceania, Africa, and Europe. The individuals whose spiritual crises follow this pattern are thus involved in an ancient process that touches the deepest foundations of the psyche.

III. Psychological Renewal Through Activation of the Central Archetype.

This type of transpersonal crisis has bee explored and described by the California psychiatrist and Jungian analyst John Weir Perry. In his clinical work with young psychotic patients, twelve of whom he saw in systematic intensive psychotherapy over long periods of time, he recognized to his surprise that the psychotic process was far from being an absurd and erratic product of pathological processes in the brain.

If sensitive support was provided, the nature of the psychopathological development was drastically transformed and what resulted was emotional healing, psychopathological development was drastically transformed and what resulted was emotional healing, psychological renewal and deep transformation of the patients' personalities. Moreover, John Perry discovered in this work that the majority of his patients manifested certain standard experiential patterns and characteristic stages if their process was not suppressed by routine psychopharmaceutic treatment.

The individuals in this type of crisis experience themselves as being in the middle of the world process, as being the center of all things, which Perry attributes to the activation of what he calls the central archetype. They are preoccupied with death and the themes of ritual killing, martydom, crucifixion, and afterlife. Another important theme is return to the beginnings of the world to creation, the original paradisiacal state, or the first ancestor.

The experiences typically focus on some cataclysmic clash of opposite forces on a global, or even cosmic level that has the quality of a sacred combat. The more mundane form of these experiences stage as protagonists capitalists and communists, Americans and Russians, the white and yellow race, secret societies against the rest of the world, and the like. The archetypal form of this conflict involves the forces of light and darkness, Christ and Antichrist or the Devil, Armeggedon, and the Apocalypse.

A characteristic element of this process is preoccupation with the reversal of opposites – cultural, ethical, political or religious beliefs, values, and attitudes. This is expressed particularly strongly in the sexual area. It involves intense misgiving in regard to the opposite sex, homosexual wishes or panic, and fear of the other sex or gender reversal. These problems find their resolution typically in the theme of the union of opposites, particularly the Sacred Marriage (hierosgamos). It is a union of a mythological nature, an archetypal fusion of the feminine and masculine aspects of one's personality. Here belongs the belief of being selected as spouse for a god or goddess, becoming a bride to Christ, being visited by the Holy Spirit as the Virgin Mary, identification with Adam and Eve, marriage of the Sun and the Moon, King and Queen, or Prince and Princess.

This process culminates in an apotheosis, an experience of being raised to a highly exalted status, either above all humans, or above the human condition altogether – becoming a world savior or messiah, a king, a president, emperor of the world or even lord of the universe. This is often associated with a sense of new birth or rebirth, the other side of the all-important theme of death. Women more frequently experience giving birth to some extraordinary child-savior, redeemer, or messiah, while men more commonly experience being born themselves. The birth of the divine child is often seen as the product of the sacred marriage.

During the time of final integration, individuals tend to draw diagrams representing the quadrated world, in which the number four plays an important role – four cardinal points, four quadrants, four rivers, or a quad-rated circle. They can also create a drama, in which four kings, four countries, or four political parties play a crucial role.

In his later books, *Far Side of Madness* and *Roots of Renewal in Myth and Madness*, Perry was able to show many uncanny parallels between the ritual drama of renewal associated with sacral kingship and the sequences in the renewal process observed in acute psychotic episodes. What existed during the archaic times of sacral kingship as externalized social forms, was thus later internalized and has become inner images and processes of contemporary individuals.

IV. Psychic Opening

Transpersonal crisis of this type is characterized by striking accumulation of instances of extrasensory perception (ESP) and other parapsychological manifestations. In acute episodes of such a crisis, the individual can be literally flooded by extraordinary paranormal experiences. Among these are various forms of out-of-body phenomena (OOB); one can experience detaching from the body and observing oneself from a distance or from above. It is not uncommon to accurately witness in an OOB state events happening in another room of the building or in a remote location. This phenomenon has been repeatedly described by thanatologists in individuals facing death (Raymond Moody, Kenneth Ring, Michael Sabom), but here it occurs without the element of vital threat.

Many mystical schools and spiritual traditions describe emergence of paranormal abilities as a common and particularly tricky stage of consciousness evolution. It is considered essential not to become fascinated by the new abilities and interpret them in terms of one's own uniqueness. The danger of what Jung called "inflation of the ego" is probably greater here than with any other type of spiritual crisis.

V. Emergence of a Karmic Pattern

In a fully developed form of this type of transpersonal crisis, the individual experiences dramatic sequences that seem to be occurring in a different temporal or spatial context - in another historical period and another country. These exper ances can be quite realistic and are accompanied by st ong negative or positive emotions and intense physical sensations. The person typically has a conviction of retrieving these events from memory – reliving episodes from his or her own previous incarnations. In addition, specific aspects of such sequences suddenly seem to throw new light on various emotional, psychosomatic, and interpersonal problems of the person's present life, which were previously obscure and incomprehensible.

Kamic experiences of this kind seem to be frequently connected with simultaneous or alternately reliving of biological birth. This occurs with characteristic patterning; birth sequences involving certain specific emotions and physical sensations tend to be linked with past life themes with the same or similar elements.

When the individual's resistance against the emerging karmic material is strong – which is common in a culture for whom the concept of reincarnation is alien – it is possible to experience a variety of strange emotions, physical sensations, and distortions in interpersonal relations without confronting and recognizing the karmic pattern that underlies them. We have encountered in our workshops a number of people who relived and resolved in an experiential session with breathing, music, and body work a karmic pattern, the elements of which had been plaguing them for months in everyday life.

Full experience and good integration of past life sequences has typically dramatic therapeutic effects. Emotional, psychosomatic and interpersonal problems can be drastically alleviated or disappear after a powerful karmic experience. For this reason, therapists should recognize this phenomenon and utilize it, irrespective of their own belief system or the historical truth of such sequences.

VI. Possession States

This transpersonal crisis can occur in the context of experiential psychotherapy, a psychedelic session, or as a spontaneous development in the life of an individual. It happens that during experiential work with or without drugs, the nature of the process suddenly changes dramatically. The face of the client can become cramped and takes the form of a mask of evil, the eyes assume a wild expression, the hands and the body show bizarre contortions, and the voice has an uncanny quality.

When this condition is allowed to develop fully, the session can bear a striking resemblance to exorcist seances in primitive cultures or medieval exorcisms of the Christian church.

The resolution of this problem requires support from people who are not afraid of the uncanny nature of the experiences involved and who can facilitate full emergence and exteriorization of the archetypal pattern. The resolution often happens after dramatic sequences of choking, projectile vomiting, or frantic motor behavior with temporary loss of control. With good support, experiences of this kind can be extremely liberating and therapeutic.

Being an initial attempt at classification in a complex territory which has not been given adequate attention in the West, the above outline is rough and sketchy. However, we hope that even in this form it will be of use to individuals undergoing transpersonal crisis and to those interested in offering assistance.

In conclusion, we would like to recommend good sources of information about specific types of transpersonal crisis for those readers who would like to explore them in greater depth. Please contact SEN-CITP for a bibliography.

Soteria: An Alternative to Hospitalization For Schizophrenics

A. Menn, A.C.S.W., L. Mosher, M.D.

Difficulties that we encounter with the treatment of psychosis in hospital settings provided a major impetus for the establishment of Soteria, a home where schizophrenics who would otherwise have been hospitalized live through their psychosis with a nonprofessional staff.

Background

Hospitals – even well-staffed "progressive" ones – invariably have institutional characteristics that create barriers to establishing the types of relationships which could maximally facilitate the process of recovery from psychosis. The "barrier" characteristics to which we refer (present to varying degrees in different settings) are of four kinds.

Theoretical Model – Although a variety of other models may be mixed in, or explicitly avowed, most psychiatric wards function primarily within a medical model. Doctors have final authority and decision-making powers; medications are accorded primary therapeutic value and used extensively; the person is seen as having a disease, with attendant disability and dysfunction that are to be "treated" and "cured"; and labeling and its consequences, objectification and stigmatization, are almost inevitable.

In contrast, at Soteria (from the Greek, salvation or deliverance) the primary focus is on growth, development, and learning. The staff are to "be with" the patients, or "residents" as we call them, to facilitate these processes insofar as they can. They share decision-making powers and responsibility with residents. They are not there either to treat or to cure the residents. Medications are infrequently used. Although we have no quarrel with the demonstrated heuristic value of the medical model, we do believe its application to psychiatric disorders can have unfortunate (and unintended) consequences for individual patients. We are not proposing an alternative model, however, because we know of none that encompasses enough of what we know about schizophrenia. We do propose an alternative attitude or stance. Basically, we advocate a phenomenological approach to schizophrenia – that is, an attempt to understand and share the psychotic person's experience without judging, labeling, or derogating it.

Size – Most psychiatric hospital wards have at least 20 patients. Thus, the staff-plus-patient group is apt to be 40 to 60. But for severely disorganized persons, a social reference group of no more than 12 to 15 persons is especially important. We believe a group of this size, when combined with a homelike atmosphere, maximizes the possibility of the disorganized person's getting to know and trust a new environment and to find a surrogate family in it. At the same time, it minimizes the labeling and stigmatization process. This number is, interestingly, about the maximum number of persons in one extended-family household, or in a single commune, and is also the upper limit for members in small task groups for group therapy and experimental psychology. Thus, rather than being a 20-bed ward, Soteria is a home that sleeps 8 to 10 comfortably, with six beds occupied by residents and two by staff.

Social Structure – Social structure interacts closely with size. To function effectively, every organization, large or small, needs structure; and generally speaking, the larger the organization, the greater the structure. Unfortunately, more elaborate structures have aspects that impinge negatively on persons undergoing psychotic disorganization – inflexibility, reliance on authority, institutionalization of roles, and decision-making power that resides in the hierarchy, outside patient's purview. Those at the bottom of the hierarchy feel relatively powerless, irresponsible, and dependent. Because of these negative aspects, at Soteria we attempt to be as un-structured as is commensurate with adequate function. Structure that develops to meet functional needs is dissolved if the need is not a continuing one. There is no institutionalized method of dealing with a particular occurrence. For example, overt aggressive acts are dealt with in a variety of ways, including strict limit-setting, depending on a myriad of variables which affect the situation. In most settings, in contrast, aggression is dealt with, almost automatically, by medication.

Medication – We live in an overmedicated, too frequently drug-dependent culture despite ambivalence which is resolved by creating two categories of drugs:

good ones like alcohol and bad ones like LSD. Our society is basically prodrug. Psychiatry's attitude is no different from that of the wider social context; we are all looking for the magical answer from a pill. The antipsychotic drugs have provided psychiatrists with real substance for their magical-cure fantasy applied to schizophrenia. But, as is the case with most such exaggerated expectations, the fantasy is better than the reality. After two decades, it is now clear that the phenothiazines do not cure schizophrenia. It is also clear that they have serious, sometimes irreversible toxicities[4] that recovery may be impaired by them in at least some schizophrenics,[6,17] and that they have little effect on longterm psychosocial adjustment.[15] These criticisms do not deny their extraordinary helpfulness in reducing and controlling symptoms, shortening hospital stays, and revitalizing interest in schizophrenia. One aim of the Soteria project is to seek a viable informed alternative to the overuse of these drugs and excessive reliance on them, often to the exclusion of psychosocial measures. We use them infrequently and when prescribed they are kept primarily under the individual resident's (patient's) control; that is, the patient is asked to monitor his or her responses to the drug very carefully, to give us feedback so we can adjust dosage, and after a trial period of two weeks he or she is given a major role in determining whether or not the drug will continue to be used.

Soteria is a reaction to criticisms of existing facilities in each of the four areas mentioned above. Much of what is involved in the program, however, is based on the positive contributions of a variety of other researchers, clinicians, and theorists. In fact, we have come to recognize that no single element of the Soteria program is new; their combination in one setting is what we believe unique. Some of Soteria's roots are to be found in: the era of moral treatment in American psychiatry[2], the tradition of intensive interpersonal intervention in schizophrenia,[5, 20] the therapists who have described growth from psychosis,[11, 16] the current group of psychiatric heretics[10, 21] and descriptions of the development of psychiatric disorder in response to life crisis.[1, 9]

Research Design

Although our research design is not the primary focus of this paper, a brief outline of it is necessary to understand the findings to be cited here. The basic design is a comparative-outcome study of two matched cohorts of first-admission, unmarried, carefully diagnosed schizophrenic patients between 16 and 30 years of age, deemed in need of hospitalization and followed for two years after admission. Both experimental and control patients are obtained from a large screening facility (600 new patients a month) that is part of a community mental health center. Patients who meet the research criteria are assigned on a consecutively admitted, space-available basis to either the experimental group or the control group.

The selection criteria are designed to provide us with a relatively homogeneous sample of individuals diagnosed schizophrenic, "at risk" for prolonged hospitalization and/or chronic disability (early onset and being unmarried both predispose to chronic care).[19] In addition to its value in homogenizing our sample, our elimination of individuals with extensive previous hospitalization reflects our wish not to deal with the learned patient role before actually involving the person as him or herself in the Soteria program. We recognize that these criteria limit our study's generalizability, but we feel that the advantages of relative homogeneity outweigh the disadvantage of more limited generalizability when it is possible to study only a relatively small number of subjects.

Control patients are admitted to the wards of the community mental health center where they receive "usual" treatment. Experimental patients, on the other hand, are treated at Soteria House. A battery of tests is used to assess both patient groups from a variety of points of view; psychiatric (diagnosis, type of onset, paranoid/nonparanoid status, symptom pattern), ward and house staff (behavior and improvement ratings), family (perception of behavior and personality characteristics), and self-rating (social and work functioning, attitude toward illness, and the like). Patients are followed at 6-month intervals for 2 years through psychiatric, family, and self ratings. All psychiatric assessments (baseline, discharge, and follow-up) are conducted by an independent evaluation team. Because the experimental treatment program is specifically designed to enhance psychosocial functioning, our postdischarge assessments address this area in particular. Because of the very different use of neuroleptics, we did not expect symptomatology (or readmission rates) to be preferentially affected by the experimental program.

The rationale and methodology of the research design has been published in detail elsewhere.[12]

The Program

Soteria is a 1915-vintage 12-room house located on a busy street in a "transitional" neighborhood of a city in the San Francisco Bay area. Bordering Soteria on one side is a nursing home and on the other a two-family home. The neighborhood has a mixture of businesses, medical facilities (a general hospital is one block away), single-family homes, and small apartments (usually homes that have been remodeled for this purpose). It is a designated poverty area inhabited by a mixture of college students, lower-income families, and former state hospital patients. Some 15-20 percent of residents in the area are Mexican-American, and there is a sprinkling of blacks.

Primarily because of licensing laws, the house may accommodate only 6 residents at one time, although as many as 10 persons can sleep there comfortably. There are 6 paid nonprofessional staff plus the project director and a quarter-time project psychiatrist. One or two new residents are admitted each month. In general, two of our specially trained nonprofessional regular staff, a man and a woman, are on duty at any one time. In addition, one or more volunteers are usually present, especially in the evening. Most staff work 36-48 hour shifts to provide themselves the opportunity to relate continuously to "spaced-out" (their term) residents over a relatively long period of time. Staff and residents share responsibility for household maintenance, meal preparation, and cleanup. Persons who are not "together" are not expected to do an equal share of the work. Over the long term, staff do more than their share and will step in to assume responsibility if a resident cannot do a task to which he has agreed. The project director acts as friend, counselor, supervisor, and object for displaced angry feelings by staff, whereas our part-time project psychiatrist supervises the staff and is seen as a stable, reassuring presence (in addition to his formal medicolegal responsibilities).

Although staff vary somewhat in how they see their roles, they generally view what psychiatry labels a "schizophrenic reaction" as an altered state of consciousness in an individual who is experiencing a crisis in living. Simply put, the altered state involves personality fragmentation, with the loss of a sense of self. In this state "beyond reason," modalities of experience merge, the inner and outer worlds become difficult to distinguish, and mystical sensations are experienced. Often the individual's terror at their altered state is reinforced by the intense fear he or she arouses in others, whose own sanity is challenged by his or her seemingly inexplicable behavior.

Few clinicians would disagree with a description of the evolution of psychosis as a process of fragmentation and disintegration. But at Soteria House, the disruptive psychotic experience is also believed to have unique potential for reintegration and reconstitution if it is not prematurely aborted or forced into some psychologically straitjacketing compromise. Our view of schizophrenia implies a number of therapeutic attitudes. All facets of the psychotic experience are taken by Soteria House staff members as "real." They view the experiential and behavioral attitudes associated with the psychosis – the clinical symptoms, including irrationality, terror, and mystical experience – as extremes of basic human qualities. Because "irrational" behavior and mystical beliefs are regarded as valid and as capable of being understood, Soteria staff try to provide an atmosphere that will facilitate integration of the psychosis into the continuity of the individual's life. Thus, psychotic persons are not to be considered nonhumans, nor are they to be related to in a depersonalized way, for such an attitude would invalidate the experience. Too often, systematic and pervasive invalidation of the psychotic person's experience by his or her family and associates appears to have contributed to the development of madness in the first place.

Any truly therapeutic program should therefore minimize invalidation. When the fragmentation process is seen as valid and as having potential for psychological growth, the individual experiencing the schizophrenic reaction can be tolerated, lived with, related to, and validated, but not "treated," or used to fulfill staff needs. Limits are set if the person is clearly a danger to themself or others, rather than merely because others are unable to tolerate his or her madness. The psychotic experience is considered intelligible in terms of the nature and characteristics of the psychosocial matrix in which it developed. That premise forms part of the basis for our orientation to the patients and their families and for the goal of developing sympathetic, understanding relationships in Soteria House.

Soteria House staff members have been selected because they seem to have the potential ability to tune in to the resident's altered state of consciousness and because they have no "theory of schizophrenia" into which he or she is to be fitted, procrustean fashion.

During the acute phase of psychosis, staff members form special one-to-one or two-to-one relationships with the disorganized resident, performing a role similar to that of the LSD-trip guide. The psychotic experience is shared and reflected, so long as both residents and staff member do not experience intolerable levels of fear and anxiety. The "guide" is someone for the resident to be with, and their intense, dyadic relationship is the program's pri-mary interpersonal unit and source of control. Phenothiazines are ordinarily not used for 6 weeks. If the resident shows no change at that time and is either paranoid or has an insidious onset, chlorpromazine (300 mg per day or more) is given. Thus far only 10 percent of Soteria residents have required a therapeutic course of phenothiazines. As residents become less psychotic, they become more active participants in the family-commune scene with its attendant problems – sibling rivalry, fairness in division of work, failures to perform as expected, and the like. These problems are worked out at the level at which they occur, ranging from between two individuals to involving the entire staff-resident group.

There is minimal organized structure. Meal preparation (including menus, cooking, and cleanup) is planned and tasks assigned at the beginning of each week. All eat together between 6 and 8 each evening and there is usually one meeting of the entire staff-resident group each week. These are the only regularly organized activities. However, everyone is free to pursue other activities like pottery, painting, yoga, and independent study, and usually does. Residents do not ordinarily use any outside mental health resources while staying at Soteria.

Authority lines and roles are flexibly defined, depending on the functions to be served; for example, there are no staff-only meetings, anyone can shop for groceries, and staff are not seen as having "the answer." they are expected to be in step with residents rather than one step ahead. There is the explicit expectation that Soteria will be transitional (for staff as well), thus setting up positive expectations that residents will eventually "get it together" and leave.

Discharge is effected by informal group consensus when residents see themselves and are seen by others as "together." Reluctance to leave is dealt with directly and firmly and is almost always accompanied by an offer to help with the process. After discharge, relationships between residents and staff are maintained if the individuals concerned are interested and agreeable.

Readers of this chapter are apt to wonder what can be derived from a program like ours, assuming it is not to be duplicated in all respects for theirs. We have come to see seven ingredients of the Soteria program as critical, and would advise others to implement all of these, or as many as possible, to facilitate the treatment of newly admitted psychotic persons. They are (1) positive expectations of learning from psychosis; (2) flexibility of roles, relationships, and responses; (3) sufficient time in residence for imitation and identification with staff to occur; (4) acceptance of the psychotic person's experience of himself as valid; (5) staff's primary responsibility to "be with" the disorganized resident, and specific acknowledgment that he need not do anything; (6) great tolerance for unusual ("crazy") behavior without anxiety or a need to control it; and (7) normalization of the experience of psychosis.

Staff

We believe that relatively untrained, psychologically unsophisticated persons can assume a phenomenological stance toward psychosis more easily than can such highly trained persons as M.D.'s or Ph.D.'s because the untrained have learned no theory of schizophrenia, whether psychodyamic, organic, or a combination of both. The unsophistication allows them freedom to be themselves, to follow their visceral responses, and to be "persons" with the psychotic individuals. Highly trained mental health professionals tend to lose this freedom in favor of a more cognitive, theory-based, learned response that may invalidate a patient's experience of him – or herself if the professional's theory-based behavior is not congruent with the patient's felt needs. Professionals may also use their theoretical knowledge defensively when confronted, in an unstructured setting, with anxiety-provoking behaviors of acute psychotics. This pattern of response is not so readily available to our unsophisticated nonprofessional therapists, nor is it reinforced by a professional degree with its status and power.

We believe the ingredients critical to the success or failure of Soteria are the characteristics and attitudes of its staff and the types of relationships developed between staff and residents. New staff are selected from a pool of candidates by the current staff-resident group in consultation with the project director. The candidates comprise persons who have heard, usually by word of mouth, about Soteria and who come because they want an opportunity to relate to unmedicated, "spaced out" individuals. Serious candidates are asked to work first as volunteers; some move into Soteria House to live, while others spend a day or more in the house each week. This process accomplishes two objectives: First, the candidate learns the principles of "being with" a resident by apprenticeship to an experienced staff person. Second, it allows the staff-resident group to get to know him well. Over time, these allow both the candidate and the house members to select each other based on experience.

The kinds of people who choose to work at Soteria are those who want neither to become part of the 9-5 business world nor to drop out and became part of the hippie scene. They are young and bright; most have attended college, but few have formal education in psychology. They can be characterized as having led intense lives in relatively few years, and as being individuals who are tough but tolerant, hard-working, energetic, and well integrated. The degree of their toughness and integration (ego strength) came as a surprise to us, because fewer than we had expected reported having experienced crises of psychotic proportions. None of the crises they did experience were labeled and treated. We also expected that many would have had extensive experience with psychedelic drugs, but that was not the case. Like most Californian youth, they have tried various drugs, but did not adopt drugs as a lifestyle. Their current use of intoxicants of any type is minimal.

In exploring the reasons for these two unexpected findings, we found a very interesting pattern; all but one of their families of origin were "problem" families. Psychiatrists reading the staff's autobiographies might well predict serious psychological problems for may of them. Instead, our staff seem to be examples of invulnerable children raised in difficult situations.

In attempting to discern the reasons for their invulnerability, we found that they had not been so intimately entwined with the psychopathologic parent as was a sibling, usually older. (Significantly, none of our staff are first-born or only children.) Although our data are incomplete on this point, the siblings of several staff members appear to be significantly psychologically impaired. Interestingly, the role most often played by our staff members in their problem families was that of a somewhat neutral caretaker for the parent. That experience may have something to do with their having chosen to work at Soteria, since a comparable pattern of family life has been noted by Henry[7] for healers and by Burton[3] for psychotherapists. Stone[18] has also noted similar phenomena in psychotherapists who had unusual success with schizophrenic patients. We have published elsewhere our complete staff data and compared them with staffs of typical hospital wards.[8, 14]

Results

Sample

A total of 37 experimental and 42 control subjects met study admission criteria and were treated in the respective facilities. By the time of this analysis, 30 experimental and 33 control subjects were eligible for 2-year follow-up. By the 2-year follow-up, 4 experimental and 10 control subjects were either lost to follow-up or refused further participation in the study. Thus, 2-year psychopathological and psychosocial data are reported from 26 experimental and 23 control subjects. Data are reported as percentages (with sample sizes at the top of each table) because we were not able to obtain 2-year data from every subject not lost to follow-up.

Baseline Assessment

There are no significant differences between the experimental and control groups on a total of 24 demographic, psychopathologic, and psychosocial variables examined on admission.

Resource Utilization

Initial Residential Care – Experimental subjects stayed significantly longer on their initial admission and less often received antipsychotic medications (Table 1). During the initial 6 weeks, no Soteria patient received antipsychotic drugs. Three subjects received them later in their stays. All control subjects received neuroleptics while hospitalized; doses averaged 730 mg per day of chlorpromazine equivalents.

Table 1
Initial Residential Care

	Experimental	Control
Length of stay: Mean ± S.D.	166 ± 142	28 + 48
Median	142 days	15 days
Neuroleptic Drug Treatment †	8% ††	100%
Average dose in chlorpromazine equivalents	660 mg/day	730 mg/day

†   Two weeks or more of antipsychotic medication at a level >300 mg/day
†† No experimental subjects received neuroleptic drugs during their initial six weeks

Table 2

Resource Utilization After Discharge

	Exper. (%)	Control (%)	Exact Prob. †
Neuroleptic drug Treatment: Cumulative to 2 years after admission	(N=23)	(N=21)	.00001
Continuous	4	43	
Intermittent ††	30	52	
Occasional	9	4	
None	57		
Other mental health contact: Cumulative to 2 years	(N=22)	(N=22)	
Any contact	59	100	.0007
Outpatient therapy	45	100	.0001
Day/night care ‡	19	41	.04
Total days/nights ‡	110	1.215	

†   Exact probability for a 2x2 contingency table.
‡   Includes readmissions to original treatment facilities as well as other psychiatric hospitals.
†† At least two weeks of continuous medication.

Readmissions – Over the 2-year follow-up, control subjects had more readmissions (67 vs. 53%) but the differences do not quite reach the .05 level of significance.

Outpatient Care After Initial Discharge

Neuroleptics. As may be seen in Table 2, over the 2-year period there were striking differences in neuroleptic drug use in the two groups. More than 50 percent of experimental subjects never received any psychotropic drugs while 43 percent of the control subjects were maintained on them.

Other outpatient care. – Table 2 indicates that control subjects more often used and consumed many more days of day or night care and outpatient therapy. Interestingly, about 40 percent of experimental subjects had no contact whatever with the regular mental health system.

Table 3
Psychosocial Adjustment: Employment

	Experi-mental (%)	Control (%)	Exact Probability†
Prior to admission	(N=36)	(N=28)	
Full-time ††	64	64	
Part-time	19	21	1.0
Not working	17	14	
Two years after admission	(N=20)	(N=19)	0.64
Full-time ††	35	21	
Part-time	45	58	
Not working	20	21	
Occupational Level ‡	2.71 ± .56	2.33 ± .49	

† Exact probability for RxC contingency table (that is, the probability of obtaining a table as probable as, or less than, the given table).

†† Full-time category includes patients attending school on a full-time basis.

‡ Significant intergroup difference $p > .05$.

Two-Year Outcome Data

Psychopathology – Although not a major focus of this paper, at 2 years overall levels and profiles of psychopathology, as rated by the Inpatient Multidimensional Psychiatric Scale (IMPS), were not

215

significantly different between the groups. Both groups showed significant and comparable reduction in psychopathology over the 2-year period.

Psychosocial Adjustment –

Employment (Table 3). – Two aspects of working are reported: overall occupational level as rated on a three-point scale (2 = fallen, 3 = same, 4 = risen) and amount of time working. There are no significant intergroup differences between the groups in percent of subjects working full- or part-time at 2 years after admission. Experimental subjects, however, had significantly higher occupational levels.

Living arrangements and friendships (Table 4). – Many more experimental subjects were living alone or with peers (that is, not at home with their families) at 2 years after admission, accounting for overall differences found. A four-point scale is used to rate how many friends patients have and how often they are seen (0 = no friends and social membership, 3= many friends and social memberships). There is a consistent nonsignificant trend favoring the experimental group on this variable.

One other preliminary result is of interest. The cost of the initial six months of care in both systems (Soteria and the "usual" state - and county-financed one) is almost exactly the same – $4,400.[13]

216

Table 4
Psychosocial Adjustment: Living Arrangements

	Exper- imental (%)	Control (%)	Exact Probabil- ity†
Prior to admission With parents/ relatives Independently †† Board and care, etc.	(N=37) 68 30 3	(N=39) 62 36 3	 .81
Two years after admission W/parents/rel. Independently †† Board and care, etc. Soteria/hospital readmission Friendships	(N=25) 28 60 12 1.95 ± .59	(N=23) 52 30 13 4 1.56 ± .92	 .03

† Exact probability for RxC contingency table (that is, the probability of obtaining a table as probable as, or less probable than, the given table).

†† Includes living alone, with peers, or with spouse and/or children.

Summary

In summary, although considerable caution should be exercised in view of the relatively small numbers of subjects studied and lack of random assignments, our data indicate that first-break schizophrenics deemed in need of hospitalization can be treated successfully by a nonprofessional staff, usually without medication, at no greater cost, in a home in the community. We have no data concerning the efficacy of this approach for long-term schizophrenics of other types of patients. It does appear, as hypothesized, that the experimental program is more effective than competent "usual" care in preserving and enhancing psychosocial adjustment in the group of subjects "at risk" for chronicity.

References

1. Birley JLT, Brown GW: Crisis and life changes preceeding the onset or relapse of acute schizophrenia: Clinical aspects. Br. J Psychiatry 116:327-333, 1970
2. Bockoven J: Moral Treatment in American Psychiatry. New York, Springer, 1963
3. Burton A: The adoration of the patient and its disillusionment. Am J Psychoanal 29:194-204, 1969
4. Crane GE: Clinical psychopharmacology in its twentieth year. Science 181(4095): 124-128, 1973
5. Fromm-Richmann F: Notes on the development of treatment of schizophrenia by psychoanalytic psychotherapy. Psychiatry 11:263-273, 1948

6. Goldstein MJ: Premorbid adjustment paranoid status and patterns of responses to phenothiazine in acute schizophrenia. Schizoph Bull 3:24-37, 1970

7. Henry WE: Some observations on the lives of healers. Human Development 9:47-56, 1966

8. Hirschfeld R, et al: Being with madness: Personality characteristics of three treatment staffs. Hosp Community Psychiatry 28(4): 267-273, 1977

9. Holmes TH, Rahe R: The social readjustment rating scale. Journal of Psychosomatic Research 11: 213-218, 1967

10. Laing RD: The Politics of Experience. New York: Ballantine Books, 1967

11. Menninger K: Psychiatrist's World: The Selected Papers of Karl Menninger, Hall BH (ed), New York: Viking Press, 1959

12. Mosher L: Research design to evaluate psychosocial treatments of schizophrenia. Hospital and Community Psychiatry 23:229-234, 1972

13. Mosher L., Menn A., Mathews S.: Soteria: Evaluation of a home-based treatment for schizophrenia. Am J Orthopsychiatry 45(3):455-467, 1975

14. Mosher L., Reifman A, Menn A: Characteristics of nonprofessionals serving as primary therapists for acute schizophrenics, Hosp Community Psychiatry 24(6):391-396, 1973

15. Niskanen P, Achte KA: The Course and Prognosis of Schizophrenic Psychoses in Helsinki: A Comparative Study of First Admissions in 1950, 1960 and 1965. Monograph No. 4. Helsinki, Finland, Psychiatric Clinic, Helsinki University Central Hospital, 1972

16. Perry JW: Reconstitutive process in the psychopathology of the self. Ann NY Acad Sci 96:853-876, 1962
17. Rappaport M, et al: Are there schizophrenics for whom driugs may be unnecessary or contraindicated? Int. Pharmacopsychiatry 13:100-111, 1978
18. Stone MH: Therapists' personality and unexpected success with schizophrenic patients. Am J Psychother 25:543-552, 1971
19. Strauss J, et al: Premorbid adjustment in schizophrenia: Concepts, measures, and implications. Schizophr Bull 3(2):182-244, 1977
20. Sullivan HS: Schizophrenia as a Human Process. New York: Norton, 1962
21. Szasz T: The Myth of Mental Illness: Foundations of a Theory of Personal Conduct. New York: Hoeber-Harper, 1961

Schizophrenics for Whom Phenothiazines are Contraindicated or Unnecessary
Esalen Institute

The following is a review of an article, recently submitted for publication to a scientific journal, entitled "Schizophrenics for Whom Phenothiazines Are Contraindicated or Unnecessary" by M. Rappaport, K. Hopkins, K. Hall, T. Belleza, and J. Silverman. The article summarized some of the results of a three year research program with diseased psychiatric patients. Designed by Drs. Julian Silverman and Maurice Rappaport, the project was carried out on a specially created experimental ward of Agnews State Hospital in San Jose, California.

One hundred twenty-seven young male schizophrenics were examined after the onset of an acute psychotic episode and also for up to three years after discharge from the hospital study. (Female patients were not included in the study; changes in females' sensory functioning are known to occur in different phases of the menstrual cycle. This fact was presumed to make it impossible to differentiate between sensory-physiological changes due to the acute schizophrenic episode and those due to menstrual cycle changes. The results of the neurophysiological research will not be summarized in this review.) Follow-up information was obtained on 108 patients for up to thirty-six months after discharge from the project. Of this number, 55% had been assigned to placebos (unmedicated pills) while in the hospital and

45% to chlorpromzine (thorazine), a popular anti-psychotic medication. Personal interviews were conducted with 80 patients and information on 28 others was obtained either through the mail, telephone, or contact with relatives. The analyses reported here are based on the 80 patients on whom full information is available.

Patients accepted for the project met the following criteria: between 16 and 40 years of age; referred from the community mental health program with a diagnosis of schizophrenia; diagnosed as having an acute schizophrenic reaction at hospital admission on the basis of evaluation with a battery of psychiatric rating scales; having no gross adverse reaction to chlorpromazine; having had no electroshock therapy within six months preceding admission; having no gross organic impairment; no history of epilepsy; no history of drug "abuse" prior to admission; and no (or few) previous hospitalizations.

When a patient was admitted to the experimental ward he was assigned randomly to either of two treatment conditions – a chlorpromazine treatment group or a placebo treatment group. Ward personnel, psychiatric raters, and all but one of the research personnel were not told to which treatment condition patients were assigned. Periodically, staff were asked to judge which patients were on chlorpromazine. Consistently, 40 to 50 percent of the time wrong judgments were tallied, indicating that staff personnel were ignorant as to patients' actual drug status.

On the first or second day after admission to the project, two trained research personnel interviewed each patient and completed a battery of psychiatric ratings including the Brief Psychiatric Rating Scale and the Global Assessment Rating Scale. Ratings on these scales were repeated at the time of each patient's discharge. Two principal measures were used. A Severity of Illness score was derived which was a composite of the above mentioned ratings. A Clinical Change Index was derived; it represented the direction of change (improvement or worsening of symptoms) from hospitalization to discharge and from discharge to follow-up. A third measure, Overall Functional Disturbance, also was utilized.

All patients took nine tablets a day (three, three times a day). Those assigned to the chlorpromazine condition received a minimum of 300 milligrams a day. The physician could order up to 900 milligrams of chlorpromzine a day. However, he was never told by the research assistant in charge whether the patient actually received medication or placebos.

Follow-up ratings were obtained, wherever possible, at 1, 3, 6, 12, 18, 24, 30, and 36 months after discharge from the hospital project.

Nurses, attendants, and doctors on the experimental ward were specially selected. Of primary concern was their willingness to work closely and continually with even very dis-eased patients and to accept as much as possible (rather than avoid) their own fears and fantasies about madness. Ongoing intensive group-work sessions for staff focused on awareness of their own feelings and openness to the feelings of others.

Findings:

Clinical Change, Severity of Illness (SI), and Overall Functional Disturbance (OFD) scores were compared for the medicated and unmedicated groups; comparisons were made at admission, discharge, and at last follow-up.

On the Clinical Change Index, significant differences, admission to discharge, were found between placebo and chlorpromazine-drugged patients. Chlorpromazine-drugged patients tended to show greater clinical changes than placebo patients while in the hospital. Thus medicated patients showed a faster and greater symptom reduction than unmedicated patients. On the Severity of Illness and Functional Disturbance scales, no significant differences were found between the medicated and unmedicated groups, at admission or at discharge. However, at follow-up, Severity of Illness scores were significantly less for placebo patients who continued off medication than for other patients. In other words, patients given placebos who stayed off medication outside of the hospital were less dis-eased at follow-up than patients given chlorpromazine while in the hospital, regardless of whether or not the hospital medicated patients continued using medication outside of the hospital. Further, greater Functional Disturbance at follow-up tended to be found among chlorpromzinedrugged patients; Functional Disturbance was less in the placebo patients than in the medicated patients. Finally, it was found that overall, significantly fewer patients were rehospitalized who had been assigned to placebos (Table 1). This was clearly apparent among patients on placebo during the project who had not used medication in the follow-up period (Table 2).

Table 1

Number of Patients Rehospitalized in Terms of Their Initial Hospital Medication Condition †

		Rehospit-alized	Not Rehospit-alized
Random Drug Assignment While Hospitalized	Placebo	12	30
	Chlorpromazine	24	15

† Information for this analysis was available on 81 patients rather than 80.

Table 2
Rehospitalizations in Relation to Hospital and Follow-up Medication Conditions

Medication Grp. In Hospital	At Follow-Up	Number of Patients	Percent Rehosp.
Placebo	Off Medication	24	8%
Chlorpromazine	On Medication	22	73%
Placebo	On Medication	17	53%
Chlorpromazine	Off Medication	17	47%

Conclusions:

In most research with acutely dis-eased patients, the foremost criterion for evaluating them favorably is still the reduction of overt and agitated psychotic behavior. The study reviewed here suggests that this criterion may, at least in certain instances, be an erroneous and unfortunate one. A significant lessening of psychotic symptoms during hospitalization, associated with phenothiazine treatment, is not related to long terms positive re-organization. Indeed it is suggested that certain acute patients, evidencing bizarre and regressive behaviors, will get better and stay better if their dis-ease is NOT interrupted with anti-psychotic chemotherapy.

Perhaps part of the reason why a significant number of placebo patients showed long-term improvements was the ward milieu that was established during the three-year period and the staff who worked on through the project. It was already known from earlier research that patients with a positive, "integrating" attitude to their dis-ease had higher levels of post-hospital adjustment several years later than those with an "isolating" (rejecting attitude toward it. In the Agnews project, this knowledge was translated into a staff attitude and a way-of-being-in-relationship which was different form many conventional hospital settings. In effect, a "space" was evolved (in a hospital setting) in which patients were given room to express their energies in relative safety; this increased the probability for these dis-eased people to rebalance themselves.

Mysticism Goes Mainstream
Andrew Greeley

Nearly half of American adults (42%) now believe they have been in contact with someone who has died, usually a dead spouse or sibling. That's up from more than one-fourth (27%) in a previous national survey done 11 years earlier.

Still higher percentages of Americans report having had psychic experiences such as extra-sensory perception (ESP). In a new survey, two-thirds of all adults (67%) now report having experienced ESP. In 1973, it was 58% in a similar poll.

Both national surveys were done by my colleagues and me at the University of Chicago's National Opinion Research Council (NORC). I became interested in what psychologists call "paranormal" experiences back in the '70s, when I began to realize how many people have them (even if they don't tell anyone).

It may well be, as Shirley MacLaine argues in the next article ("Shirley MacLaine's Spiritual Dance"), that the incidence of such experiences is rising fast. But I favor a different explanation: Partly because of her and others, millions are less afraid to talk about the experiences.

I've had no vested interest, religious or sociological, in the metaphysical reality of these experiences. I am a sociologist and novelist. I am also a parish priest, as suggested by my current book, *Confessions of a Parish Priest*. The Roman Catholic Church of this era is profoundly skeptical of paranormal phenomena. So am I. I doubt, for example, that the contact-with-the-dead experiences can ever be "scientifically" validated. But even though I've never had a psychic or mystical experience myself, most Americans have. We saw this in our first study in 1973 and in data from a repeat survey we have just analyzed.

Our new results, published here for the first time, show a clear trend: More people than ever say they've had such experiences. Other surveys confirm the trend (see "Mystical Americans," p. 49). And it's true whether you look at the most common forms of psychic and mystical experience, or the rarest.

Some experiences aren't too far from the ordinary, and may soon be explained by neurological or psychological processes – like *déja vu*, that eerie sense of going to a new place and feeling sure you've somehow been there before. 59% of Americans reported *déja vu* in 1973; today, the figure's 67%.

Other experiences, though, are profound. In 1973, a full 35% of Americans reported they had had a mystical experience; feeling "very close to a powerful, spiritual force that seemed to lift you out of yourself." And one-seventh of those who have had such experiences – 5% of the whole population – have literally been "bathed in light" like the Apostle Paul. These experiences go way beyond intellect, and even beyond emotion. For a fifth of those who have them, they involve "a sense of tremendous personal expansion, either psychological or physical" – a form of body mysticism.

Such paranormal experiences – by definition, lying outside the normal – are generally viewed as hallucinations or symptoms of mental disorder. But if these experiences were signs of mental illness, our numbers would show the country is going nuts. What was paranormal is now normal. It's even happening to elite scientists and physicians who insist that such things cannot possibly happen.

Indeed, the nation is living with a split between scientific belief and personal reality. For example, 30% of the Americans who do *not* believe in life after death still say they've been in personal contact with the dead. My friend John Shea, a theologian, believes that these encounters could be real and the cause, not the result, of man's tenacious belief in life after death. But as a scientist all I can vouch for is the fact that millions of Americans have such experiences.

In any case, our studies show that people who've tasted the paranormal, whether they accept it intellectually or not, are anything but religious nuts or psychiatric cases. They are, for the most part, ordinary Americans, somewhat above the norm in education and intelligence and somewhat less than average in religious involvement.

We tested people who'd had some of the deeper mystical experiences – such as being bathed in light. We began with the Affect Balance Scale of psychological well-being, a standard measure of the healthy personality. And the mystics scored at the top. Norman Bradburn, the University of Chicago psychologist who developed the scale, said no other factor has ever been found to correlate so highly.

When we reported our first NORC survey in 1973, a scientific sample of 1,467 adults, we soon discovered how nervous people can be about spirituality. Many, particularly in academia and the media, find it unthinkable that a sizable proportion of the people they see every day believe they have experiences outside the accepted limits of science. This discomfort has made it hard to carry on serious academic discussion about the mystical experiences of ordinary Americans.

I've been using my survey findings in a series of bestselling novels, beginning with *The Cardinal Sins* (Warner Books). While the incidents in my books are fictional, each is based on one or more personal interviews with people who tell their stories.

So, in *Lord of the Dance,* the heroine Noele Farrel is psychic. Annie Reilly in *Angels of September* sees her adolescent sweetheart – who'd been killed in the Hurtgen Forest battle 40 years earlier – walking along Chicago's Oak Street Beach. In this year's *Patience of a Saint,* Redmond Peter Kane is bowled over by an intense mystical experience on Wacker Drive as he walks by the ice-green 333 Wacker Drive Building. In the upcoming *Rite of Spring*, Brendan Ryan walks into his room in a Grand Beach summer home and finds his murdered wife, still lovely, calmly waiting for a chat with him. She has been guided to his room by Jackie Curran, a five-year-old who's psychic.

Some readers (and critics especially) raise a protest: Such events don't happen. They shouldn't be in fiction. Perhaps out of Celtic perversity, I disagree. To pretend that such perceptions do not occur to ordinary people in everyday life is like a Victorian novelist pretending that sexual intercourse does not occur. Either sham is, to say the least, nonscientific if not inhuman.

Despite years of attempts to study paranormal phenomena, there's been a scientific iron curtain raised against serious research on these experiences. But a crack in it opened a few years ago. Researchers in Japan and Wales, then in England, began to report on contact with the dead, especially among widowers in nursing homes. A University of North Carolina team led by associate professor of family medicine P. Richard Olson found that nearly two-thirds (64%) of widows at two Asheville nursing homes had at least "once or twice felt as though they were in touch with someone who had died."

That's not surprising by itself. What *is* surprising is the vividness of the experiences. Of those who reported such contact, 78% said they saw the dead one. 50% heard, 21% touched, 32% felt the presence, 18% talked with the departed and 46% had some combination of the above. Most found the encounter helpful, not scary, but none had ever mentioned the incident to their doctors.

"It's not well known that such experiences are common, but they are," Olson says. In *Geriatrics Today*, he writes that even psychoactive drugs didn't end the "visits."

Our second NORC survey of paranormal experiences included a national sample of 1,473 adults in 1984. When I recently finished work with that data, it showed a marked increase in the number of men and women willing to report the encounters, at least in the anonymity of a polling interview. Among widows and widowers in the general population, our survey just about replicated Olson's findings in North Carolina.

We asked ourselves whether psychic and mystical beliefs cause the experience, or experience causes the belief. We turned to our national sample – this time to check for belief in life after death, intensity of religious commitment, and whether respondents envision a loving God or a judgmental one. We found, surprisingly, that many widows who experienced these visitation had not previously believed in life after death. So they were not hallucinating an image to match their beliefs (at least, not their conscious beliefs). This suggests, though it does not prove, that the experience is more likely to cause a belief in the hereafter than the other way around.

Pollster Andrew Greeley and colleagues at the University of Chicago have tracked our spiritual health since 1973. The data show that more Americans report paranormal experiences now than in the '70s ('73 results in Parentheses).

Americans Who:

Had contact with the dead (adult pop.)	(27%) 42%
Had contact with the dead (widows)	(51%) 67%
Had visions	(8%) 29%
Experienced ESP	(58%) 67%
Experienced *deja vu*	(59%) 67%
Experienced clairvoyance	(24%) 31%
Believe in life after death	(*) 73%
Believe the afterlife is Paradise	(*) 68%
Believe that after death they'll be reunited with dead loved ones	(*) 74%

*no figures available

National surveys by The Gallup Organization bolster Greeley's polls showing paranormal experiences in the USA are on the rise:

Had an unusual spiritual experience	43% ('85)
Had a near-death experience	15% ('81)
Believe in life on other planets	46% ('81)
Believe in life after death	71% ('81)
Believe in reincarnation	23% ('81)
Believe in God or a Universal Spirit	95% ('81)
Believe Jesus is God	70% ('83)
Believe in angels	67% of teenagers ('86)
Believe in heaven **	71% ('80)
Believe in hell	53% ('80)
Expect the afterlife to be boring	5% ('81)

**Of those who believe, 20% ('81) think their chances of going to heaven are excellent.

We also asked whether people who'd lost a parent or child reported contact with the dead more than people whose siblings had died – on the theory that those who'd lost closer family members would have a greater "need" to hallucinate visitations. Again, we were surprised: People who'd lost a child or parent were less likely to report contact with the dead than those who'd lost siblings.

These findings make it difficult to explain such talks with the departed as simple psychological wish-fulfillment. But one finding does give a clue to the psychology of these experiences. For widows and for people who had lost siblings alike, the major factor associated with contacting the dead was a belief in a loving God, rather than a judgmental one. Though intriguing, however, this still doesn't prove whether belief or experience comes first. Feeling contact with a dead relative could certainly change one's mind about God, and make it easier to picture a warm, loving deity.

Whatever the cause of these "visitations," our work confirms the North Carolina suggestion that these experiences are common, benign and often helpful. What has been "paranormal" is not only becoming normal in our time – it may also be health-giving.

That has not made the news welcome to the routine scientist. There's an understandable resistance to studying phenomena, however benign, whose nature we really don't understand. It would be easier, certainly, to deny that these experiences exist.

But the data show clearly that they *do* exist, that people experience them in great numbers – and that they could even change the nature of our society. What may be most significant in our studies is not that the majority of adults now report experiencing ESP, or even that nearly half feel that they have talked with the dead. A small minority, maybe under 20 million, have undergone profoundly religious moments of ecstasy. They report out-of-body trips, being bathed in light, or other encounters that transform their lives. They become profoundly trusting, convinced that something good rules in the world. Whether their number is growing or they're just now ready to tell about it, that many people capable of trust can have a lasting effect on the country.

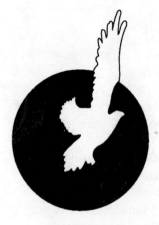

Appendix D ─────────────────

Referrals

This section is divided into four headings. 'SEN Conferences of 1985' reviews the 1985 conferences briefly and gives a brief introduction to the people who participated. 'References to Referral Networks' gives the names, addresses and phone numbers of networks who refer people to Helpers. '24 Hour Care Centers' gives the names and addresses of sanctuaries for people in crisis. 'References' is a list of books on the phenomenology of spiritual emergence which would be helpful for anyone wanting to know more about the topic.

SEN Conferences of 1985

The Spiritual Emergence Network conferences of 1985 were held for the following purposes:

1. To enhance communication between clinicians working with people in spiritual emergency.

2. To increase our understanding of diagnosis where phenomena of spiritual emergence are present.

3. To understand the role of residential treatment centers for people in spiritual emergency.

4. To understand the role of Helpers who support people in spiritual emergence and emergency.

5. To consider the elements that catalyze spiritual emergence within individuals and within collective groups.

6. To support the development of the Spiritual Emergence Network.

The conferences each focused on producing particular products. The October, 1985 conference participants collected ideas towards creating a "Training Manual" for teaching professionals and para-professionals how to work with people undergoing crises of spiritual emergence. The May, 1985 conference dedicated some intensive work toward questions of enhancing communication networking for SEN on a worldwide basis.

The participants who attended the conferences were psychologists, psychiatrists, administrators, spiritual teachers, monastics, and students of transpersonal psychology. Following is a list of these people, a short description of their work, and the topic of their talk, if they gave one.

The May,1985 Conference Participants:

Anne and Jim Armstrong: Anne is a psychic counselor who, together with her husband, Jim, teaches people how to use their intuition. They spoke on "Psychic Opening and Spiritual Emergence."

Angeles Arrien, M.A.: symbol consultant, anthropologist and teacher of universal symbols and Shamanism. Arrien spoke about "Universal Symbols in Spiritual Emergence."

Dominie Cappadonna, Ph.D.: teacher of transpersonal psychology, healer, and tour guide. Cappadonna spoke about "Global Spiritual Emergence ."

Susanna Davila, Ph.D.: administrator of the Transpersonal Counseling Center at the Institute of Transpersonal Psychology, supervisor for the Spiritual Emergence Network.

Christina Grof and Stanislav Grof, M.D.: authors and founders of SEN; S. Grof has done over 20 years of research in the area of consciousness studies. Dr. Grof dialogued with Lama Sogyal Rinpoche on the subject of "Diagnosing Spiritual Emergency." He and Christina also dialogued with the Hendricks on the similarities and differences in their respective work with the body using the breath.

Gay Hendricks, Ph.D., Kathlyn Hendricks, Ph.D., A.D.T.R.: therapists and teachers of transpersonal breathwork, the Hendricks spoke on "Spiritual Emergence/Emergency as a Somatic Experience."

Voyce Hendrix and Betty Dahlquist: administrators of California Association of the Social Rehabilitation Agencies. They participated in the discussion led by Telles on "Organizing Residential Treatment Centers and Educational Models for Training Counselors."

Charles Lonsdale, M.A.: (then) administrator of SEN.

Francis Lu, M.D.: psychiatrist and professor at the University of California. Dr. Lu spoke on his work and dialogued with Ralph Metzner on "The Use of Pharmaceuticals for people in Spiritual Emergency."

Ralph Metzner, Ph.D.: psychologist, author, administrator at California Institute of Integral Studies. Metzner spoke on "Diagnosing Spiritual Emergence" and dialogued with Dr. Lu on "The Use of Pharmaceuticals for People in Spiritual Emergency."

Lama Sogyal Rinpoche: an honored spiritual teacher from Tibet, spoke on "Diagnosing Spiritual Emergency."

Sharon Solfvin, M.A.: administrator at J.F.K. University and counselor.

Lawrence Telles, Ph.D.: academic philosopher, coordinator of invited conferences on 'Psychosocial Alternatives to Traditional Psychiatric Care.' Telles spoke about his work "Organizing Residential Treatment Centers and Educational Models for Training Counselors."

Bryan Wittine, Ph.D.: transpersonal therapist and (then) administrator at J.F.K.University's School of Consciousness Studies. Wittine spoke about "Transpersonal Therapy and the Dark Night of the Soul."

Frances Vaughan, Ph.D.: professor of transpersonal psychology, author, and psychologist. Vaughan spoke about "Transpersonal Psychotherapy and Ego Development."

Karen Paine-Gernee: educator and counselor, spoke about "Spiritual Emergence and Adult Children of Alcoholics."

Mitchell May, M.A.: healer and educator. May spoke about "Physical Emergencies which Precipitate Spiritual Emergence."

241

Dick Price: (then) president of Esalen Institute.

Father Thomas: Benedictine monk, dialogued with Brother David and Dick Price on "Communities which Foster Spiritual Emergence."

Brother David Steindl-Rast: Benedictine monk, author and lecturer on Eastern and Western Spirituality. Brother David dialogued on "Communities which Foster Spiritual Emergence."

Peggy Taylor and Paul Taylor, Ph.D.: (then) coordinators for SEN at Esalen, and transpersonal counselors.

SEN Volunteers- **Emma Bragdon, M.A.; William Brater, M.A.; Eric Lehrman, M.A.; Megan Nolan, Ph.D.; David Rasch, M.A.**

The October, 1985 SEN Conference Participants:

Jamie Baraz: spiritual teacher within the Vipassana community. Baraz spoke on "Managing Spiritual Crises in Spiritual Communities."

Mara Suzana Behlau and Roberto Zeimer: SEN Regional Coordinators from Brazil. They spoke about "Supporting Spiritual Emergence in South America."

Elizabeth Campbell, Ph.D.: moderator of the conference, (then) administrator of the External Degree program at the Institute of Transpersonal Psychology, teacher. Campbell spoke on "Networking."

Cecil Chamberlin, M.D.: psychiatrist at the Menninger Foundation, and SEN Regional Coordinator in Kansas. Dr. Chamberlin spoke about his work and "Supporting Spiritual Emergence in North America."

Susanna Davila, Ph.D.: Administrator of the Transpersonal Center and supervisor for SEN at the Institute of Transpersonal Psychology.

Christina Grof and Stanislav Grof, M.D.: founders of SEN. They spoke about "Supporting Spiritual Emergence Internationally."

Willis Harman, Ph.D.: President of the Institute of Noetic Sciences, professor at Stanford, Senior Social Scientist at Stanford Research Institute, and author. Harman spoke on "The Emerging Global Consciousness."

Michel Henry: administrator of a philanthropic organization, and teacher. Henry spoke about "Global Networking."

Frank Kretschmer, M.A.: Regional Coordinator for SEN in Germany, transpersonal therapist. Kretschmer spoke with Pennington on "Supporting Spiritual Emergence in Europe."

Alicia Mayo: SEN Regional Coordinator in Mexico, counselor and educator. Mayo spoke on "Curanderismo: A Healing System of Mexico" and her work supporting spiritual emergence in Mexico.

Megan Nolan, Ph.D.: (then) Administrator of SEN. Nolan gave current information on SEN.

Judith Orloff,M.D.: psychiatrist and regional coordinator for SEN in southern California.

George Pennington: SEN regional coordinator in Germany, transpersonal counselor, administrator of a residential treatment facility in Germany, "Esse". Pennington spoke on "Supporting Spiritual Emergence in Europe."

John Perry, M.D.: psychiatrist, author, past coordinator of Diabysis- a residential treatment center in San Francisco. Dr. Perry spoke about "Residential Treatment Centers: A Model for World-Wide Use."

Dick Price: (then) president of Esalen Institute. Price dialogued with Perry on "Residential Treatment Centers."

Swami Radha: spiritual teacher from Canada. Swami Radha spoke about "Managing Spiritual Crisis in Spiritual Communities."

Aminah Raheem, Ph.D.: teacher of Jin Shin Do at Institute of Transpersonal Pschology, Transpersonal Integration Practitioner. Raheem spoke on "Identifying Crises of Spiritual Emergence and Facilitating Transformation."

Jacquelyn Small, MSSW: author, teacher, and counselor. Small talked about "Identifying Crises of Spiritual Emergence and Facilitating Trans-formation." She also led an experiential session in Holotropic Therapy.

Brother David Steindl-Rast: Benedictine monk, lecturer, and author. Brother David spoke about his experiences "Supporting Spiritual Emergence Internationally."

Peggy Taylor and Paul Taylor, Ph.D.: (then) SEN coordinators at Esalen, transpersonal counselors. Paul Taylor spoke on "The New Physics and Spiritual Emergence."

Roger Bunting: administrator of Metasystems Design Group, Inc. Bunting discussed "Networking" and, more specifically, "Metasystem Computer Technology."

Lee Sannella, M.D.: psychiatrist, opthalmologist, author. Sannella discussed "What Makes a Good Helper?"

Larry Telles, Ph.D.: academic philosopher and administrator in the field of psycho-social rehabilitation.   Telles dialogued with Perry on "Residential Treatment Centers."

SEN Volunteers: **Emma Bragdon, M.A.; David Warren, Ph.D.; Edris Head; Eric Lehrman, M.A.; Ruth Norman.**

Note: To preserve the privacy and exploratory nature of the work at the SEN conferences,1985, we decided not to make the tapes of the conferences available to the general public.   Our agreement with the participants is that none of the discussions or presentations would be quoted in publications without their prior consent.

References to Referral Networks

Following is a list of referral networks that can help educate people about spiritual emergence processes, and refer people to qualified Helpers fand Care Centers for support and/or therapy.

The Spiritual Emergence Network
250 Oak Grove Avenue
Menlo Park, CA. 94025
Telephone: 415-327-2776

John F. Kennedy University School
   of Consciousness Studies
12 Altarinda Road
Orinda, CA. 94563
Attention: Sharon Solfvin
Telephone: 415-254-0200

International Association of Near Death Studies (IANDS)
Department of Psychiatry
University of Connecticut Health Center
Farmington, Connecticut 06032

> [IANDS had to discontinue its telephone networking service in Spring,1987. They are now only taking care of correspondence dealing with research. They hope to expand their services again in the near future. IANDS is now primarily involved in NDE experience and "its implications."]

24 Hour Care Centers

Burch House
RFD #1
Littleton, NH 03561
Telephone: 603-444-6938

Pocket Ranch
PO Box 516
Geyserville, CA 95441
Telephone: 707-857-3359

Written Literature on the Phenomenology of Spiritual Emergence and Emergency.

The following books are appropriate to educate yourself further on the experiences people have had as they reach transpersonal states of consciousness. These books are also educational for clients looking for more information about transpersonal states of consciousness.

Capra, F., The Tao of Physics, Boulder, Co.: Shambhala, 1975.

Capra, F., The Turning Point, N.Y.: Simon and Schuster, 1982.

Da Free John, The Dawn Horse Testament, San Rafael, CA: Dawn Horse Press, 1985.

Dass, Ram, The Only Dance There Is, New York: Doubleday and Co., 1974.

Golas, T., The Lazy Man's Guide To Enlightenment, New York: Bantam, 1972.

Gopi Krishna, Kundalini, The Evolutionary Energy in Man, Berkeley,CA: Shambhala, 1971.

Grof, S., Beyond the Brain, Albany, NY: State University of New York Press, 1985.

Haich, E., Initiation, Palo Alto, CA:The Seed Center, 1974.

James, W., Varieties of Religious Experience, NY: Collier Books, 1961.

Keyes, K., Handbook to Higher Consciousness, Coos Bay, Oregon: Living Love Publications, 1972.

Maslow, A.H., Religions, Values, and Peak Experiences, NY: Viking Press, 1970.

Monroe, R., Journeys Out of the Body, Garden City, NJ: Doubleday, 1971.

Rama, Swami, Ajaya, Swami, and Ballentine,R., Yoga and Psychotherapy: The Evolution of Consciousness, Honesdale, PA: Himalayan International Institute, 1976.

'Revision', Journal of Consciousness and Change, Vol.8,#1,1985.

Ring, K., Heading Toward Omega, NY: William Morrow and Co., 1984.

Sannella, L., Kundalini: Psychosis or Transcendence, San Francisco: H.S. Dakin, 1976.

Small, J., Transformers: The Therapists of the Future, Marina Del Rey, CA: DeVorss and Co., 1982.

Trungpa, C., and Freemantle, F., Tibetan Book of the Dead, Berkeley, CA: Shambhala, 1975.

Walsh, R., and Vaughan, F., <u>Beyond Ego</u>, LA: Tarcher, 1980.

Weil, A., <u>The Natural Mind, a New Way of Looking at Drugs and Higher Consciousness</u>, NY: Houghton Mifflin, 1972.

White, J., <u>What is Enlightenment?</u> L.A.: Tarcher, 1984.

Wilber, K. <u>Atman Project: A Transpersonal View of Human Development</u>, Wheaton, Ill.: Theosophical Publishing House, 1980.

Yogananda, P., <u>Autobiography of a Yogi</u>, LA: Self-Realization Fellowship,1946.

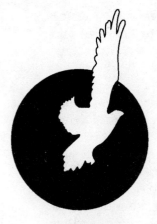

Appendix E ————————

Glossary

Atman: A level or state of consciousness described as the suchness of all states, the radically perfect integration of all prior levels of consciousness.

Bio-energy: The fundamental source that pulsates and charges the body; the root of all subjective experience, body expression (including emotion) and movement (Lowen, 1958; Kelley, 1970).

Breathwork: A therapeutic modality using amplification of breathing to energize and support the psychic /somatic homeostatic process.

Causal: A level or state of consciousness which includes direct identification with the Divine.

COEX system: System of condensed experience; intense experiences from previous personal history including birth and past-lives, which have not yet been metabolized and exist in one's psychic structure inhibiting further development to some extent (Grof,1985).

Ego: The organizing principle of the self.

Helper: A professional or paraprofessional who acts as a companion and guide to a person in spiritual emergence/ emergency.

Kundalini: The creative energy of the universe which lies dormant at the base of the human spine until activated; when activated it rises up the spine as active energy—opening, clearing, and lighting the energetic centers of the body (Mookerjee, 1982).

Psychosis: Any major disorder in which the personality is very seriously disorganized and contact with reality impaired.

Self-structure: The level or structure of consciousness attained in an individual's development. It is assumed that once a level of consciousness emerges in human development, it tends to remain in existence in the life of the individual during subsequent development (Wilber, 1984 a & b).

Spiritual emergence: The process of personal awakening into a level of perceiving and functioning that is beyond normal ego functioning. It involves having spiritual experiences and integrating these experiences into a positive framework for increased well being.

Spiritual emergency: Profound disorientation and instability that sometimes accompanies intense spiritual experiences. Spiritual emergency appears as an acute psychotic episode lasting between minutes and weeks. It has a positive, transformative outcome.

Spiritual experience: Any experience of the Subtle, Causal, or Atman levels of consciousness.

Subtle: A level or state of consciousness which includes psi phenomena, out-of-body experience, expanded sensory perceptions, and deep inspiration. It is the seat of the actual archetypes, and perceptions of God.

Transpersonal: Having to do with experiences that are beyond normal ego states, i.e. extraordinary well-being, optimal psychological health.

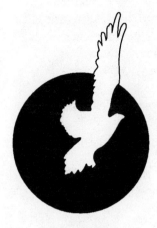

Appendix F ━━━━━━━━━━━━━

References

Allison, F. (1967). Adaptive Regression and Intense Religious Experience. <u>Journal of Nervous Mental Disorders, 145,</u> 452-463.

American Psychiatric Association (1980). <u>Diagnostic and Statistical Manual of Mental Disorders (3rd ed.)</u> Washington, D. C. : Author.

Armstrong, A. (1985, May). SEN conference.

Armstrong, A. (1986). The Challenges of Psychic Opening: A Personal Story. <u>ReVision.</u> 8 (2).

Armstrong, T. (1985). The Radiant Child. Wheaton, Ill. : Quest Books.

Baraz, J. (1985, Oct.). SEN conference.

Bly, R. (1971). The Kabir Book. Boston: Beacon Press.

Boisen, A. T. (1962). The Exploration of the Inner World. NY: Harper and Brothers.

Bolen, J. (1984). seminar on "The Heroine's Journey." San Francisco: Jung Institute.

Cappadonna, D. (1985, May). SEN conference.

Chamberlin, C. (1986) Supporting Spiritual Emergence. SEN Newsletter.

Cusack, C. (1974). Transcendental Runner. In Runner's World (eds.) The Complete Runner . New York: Harper and Row, pp. 18-25.

Cucuruto, P. (1977). training seminar. San Francisco.

Dabrowski, K. (1964). Positive Disintegration. Boston: Little Brown.

Da Free John (1985). The Dawn Horse Testament. San Rafael: Dawn Horse Press.

Eliade, M. (1964). Shamanism: Archaic Techniques of Ecstasy. Bollingen Series, vol. 76. New York: Pantheon Books.

Esalen Institute (1971). Schizophrenics for whom Phenothiazines are Contraindicated or Unnecessary. Big Sur: Author.

Ferguson, M. (Ed.) (1985). Psychotherapists Report on Drugs' Clinical Outcome. Brain-Mind Bulletin 10 (8), 1&3.

Goldstein, J. (1976). The Experience of Insight. Boston: Shambhala.

Greeley, A. M. (1975). The Sociology of the Paranormal. Beverley Hills, CA: Sage.

Greeley, A. M. (1987, January-February). Mysticism goes Mainstream. American Health.

Greer, G. (1983). MDMA: A new Psychotropic Compound and its Effects in Humans. Santa Fe, NM: Author

Grof, S. (1980). LSD Psychotherapy. Pomona, CA: Hunter House.

Grof, S. (1985, May). SEN conference.

Grof, S. (1985). Beyond the Brain. Albany, NY: State University of New York Press.

Grof, S. & Grof, C. (1985). Forms of Spiritual Emergency. SEN Newsletter, 1 (3). Menlo Park, CA: ITP.

Grof, S. & Grof, C. (1986). Spiritual Emergency: The Understanding and Treatment of Transpersonal Crises. ReVision. 8 (2), 7-20.

Harman, W. (1985, Oct.). SEN conference.

Hendricks, G. (1985, May). SEN conference.

Hendricks, K. (1985, May). SEN conference.

Hood, R. (1974). Psychological Strength and the Report of Intense Religious Experience. Journal of the Scientific Study of Religion. 13, 65-71.

Huxley, A. (1977). In Horowitz & Palmer, (eds.) Moksha. Los Angeles: Tarcher.

Jackson, E. (1984). training seminar. Berkeley.

James, W. (1961). The Varieties of Religious Experience. New York: Collier-Macmillan Ltd.

Johnstone, R. (1973). A Ketamine trip. Anaesthesiology. 39, 460-461.

Jung, C. G. (1961). Memories, Dreams and Reflections. New York: Random House.

Jung, C. G. (1968). Analytic Psychology: Its Theory and Practice. New York: Random House.

Kelly, C. (1971). Education in Feeling and Purpose. Ojai, CA: Radix Institute.

Kennett, J. (1982). Teaching seminar. Institute of Transpersonal Psychology.

Krishna, Gopi (1971). Kundalini:The Evolutionary Energy in Man. Boston: Shambhala.

Krishna, Gopi (1975). Science and Kundalini. a paper presented at the seminar on Yoga, Science and Man. New Delhi.

Laing, R. D. (1972). Metanoia: Some experiences at Kingsley Hall, in Ruitenbeek (Ed.), Going Crazy (pp.11-21) New York: Bantam.

Lievegoed, B. (1979). Phases: Crisis and Development in the Individual. London: Rudolf Steiner Press.

Lindberg, A. M. (1955). Gift from the Sea. New York: Pantheon.

Lowen, A. (1958). The Language of the Body. New York: MacMillan.

Lowen, A. & Lowen, L. (1977). The Way to Vibrant Health. New York: Harper and Row.

Lukoff, D. (1985). Diagnosis of Mystical Experiences with Psychotic Features. Journal of Transpersonal Psychology. 17 (2), 155-181.

Lukoff, D. & Everest, H. (1985). The Myths of Mental Illness. The Journal of Transpersonal Psychology. 17 (2), 123-153.

MacLaine, S. (1984). <u>Dancing in the Light</u>. New York: Bantam.

Maslow, A. (1971). <u>The Farther Reaches of Human Nature</u>. New York: Viking Press.

McGlashan, A. (1970). <u>The Savage and Beautiful Country</u>. London: Chatto and Windus.

Mosher, L. and Menn, A. (1979). Soteria: An Alternative to Hospitalization for Schizophrenics. <u>New Direction for Mental Health Services</u>, <u>1</u>, San Francisco: Jossey-Bass, pp. 73-84.

Perry, J. (1974). <u>The Far Side of Madness</u>. N. J. : Prentice-Hall.

Perry, J. (1986). Spiritual emergence and renewal. <u>ReVision</u>. <u>8</u> (2), 33-38.

Pirsig, R. (1974). <u>Zen and the Art of Motorcycle Maintenance</u>. New York: William Morrow and Co.

Platt, J. (1983). in Russell, P., <u>The Global Brain</u>. Los Angeles: Tarcher, p. 74.

Raheem, A. (1985, October). SEN conference.

Rama, Swami, & Ballentine, R. & Ajaya, Swami (1976). <u>Yoga and Psychotherapy</u>, Honesdale, PA: Himalayan Institute.

Ring, K. (1980). <u>Life at Death</u>. New York: Quill.

Ring, K. (1984). Heading Towards Omega. New York: William Morrow.

Rogo, D. (1984), Ketamine and the Near-Death Experience. Anabiosis-The Journal of Near Death Studies 4 (1), 87-96.

Russell, P. (1983). The Global Brain. Los Angeles: Tarcher.

Sannella, L. (1976). Kundalini: Psychosis or Transcendence?. San Francisco: H.S. Dakin Co.

Silverman, J. (1971). A Paradigm for the Study of Altered States of Consciousness. Journal of Psychedelic Drugs. 3 (2), 89-103.

Small, J. W. (1985). Floodtide. San Francisco: J. W. Small.

Speeth, K. (1982). On Psychotherapeutic Attention. Journal of Transpersonal Psychology, 14 (2), 141-160.

Stein, M. (Ed.) (1984). Jungian Analysis. Boulder: Shambhala.

Steindl-Rast, D. (1985, May). SEN conference.

Strassman, R. (1984). Adverse Reactions to Psychedelic Drugs: A Review of the Literature. Journal of Nervous and Mental Disease, 172 (10), 577-595.

Suzuki, S. (1970). Zen Mind, Beginner's Mind. New York: Weatherhill.

Thomas, L. & Cooper, P. (1977). Incidence and Psychological Correlates of Intense Spiritual Experiences. paper presented at East Psychological Meeting, Boston.

Toufexis, A. (1985, June 10). A Crackdown on Ecstasy. Time Magazine, p. 64.

Vaughan, F. (1985, May). SEN conference.

Vaughan, F. (1986). The Inward Arc. Boston: Shambhala.

Walsh, R. & Vaughan, F. (1980). Beyond Ego. Los Angeles: Tarcher Press.

Weil, A. (1972). The Natural Mind. New York: Houghton Mifflin.

White, J. (Ed.) (1984). What is Enlightenment? Los Angeles: Tarcher Press.

Wilber, K. (1980). The Atman Project. Wheaton, Ill.: Theosophical Publishing House.

Wilber, K. (1984). The Developmental Spectrum and Psychopathology. Part I , Journal of Transpersonal Psychology. 16 (1), 75-118.

Wilber, K. (1984). The Developmental Spectrum and Psychopathology. Part II, Journal of Transpersonal Psychology. 16 (2), 137-166.

Wittine, B. (1985, May). SEN conference.

Yogananda, P. (1946). <u>Autobiography of a Yogi.</u> Los Angeles: Self-Realization Press.

Young, V. (1983). <u>Working with Death: A Trainer's Manual.</u> (doctoral dissertation, ITP).

Ordering Information

To order additional copies of **The Sourcebook For Helping People in Spiritual Emergency** . . .

Send order to: Lightening Up Press
885 No. San Antonio Rd.
Suite 'R'
Los Altos, California 94022
(408) 688-4745

Please include:
Name _____

Address _____

_____

Phone _____

Price/Copy _____ $11.95 X _____

No. of Copies _____

Subtotal _____

6.5% Sales Tax for
California Residents _____ + _____

Postage and Handling
$2.00 Per Copy _____ + _____

TOTAL _____

Make Checks
Payable To: Lightening Up Press

Bulk orders may be purchased at a reduced rate.